MY BRIDGE WAS COLLAPSING:
Surviving While Caring for a Spouse with Dementia

JANE GRUDT

EDITED BY JOY SEPHTON

My Bridge Was Collapsing:
Survival While Caring for a Spouse with Dementia

© Copyright 2024 Jane Grudt

All rights reserved. No part of this publication may be reproduced, distributed, or transmitted in any form or by any means, including photocopying, recording, or other electronic or mechanical methods, without the prior written permission of the author, except in the case of brief quotations embodied in critical reviews and certain other noncommercial uses permitted by copyright law.

Although the author has made every effort to ensure that the information in this book was correct at press time, the author does not assume and hereby disclaim any liability to any party for any loss, damage, or disruption caused by errors or omissions, whether such errors or omissions result from negligence, accident, or any other cause.

Adherence to all applicable laws and regulations, including international, federal, state, and local governing professional licensing, business practices, advertising, and all other aspects of doing business in the US, Canada, or any other jurisdiction, is the sole responsibility of the reader and consumer.

The author does not assume any responsibility or liability whatsoever on behalf of the consumer or reader of this material. Any perceived slight of any individual or organization is purely unintentional.

The resources in this book are provided for informational purposes only. They should not be used to replace the specialized training and professional judgment of a health care or mental health care professional.

The author cannot be held responsible for the use of the information provided within this book. Please always consult a trained professional before making any decision regarding treatment of yourself or others.

Cover sketch by Jane Grudt

For more information, email: jgrudt@gmail.com

ISBN: 979-8-9904827-0-8 paperback

ISBN: 979-8-9904827-1-5 ebook

Dedication

This book is dedicated to the memory of my loving husband, Louis Grudt, now in the care of his Heavenly Father.

We have been blessed with a wonderful son and his family:

Paul and Megan Grudt, Malayna, and Stella; our sisters, Paula Grudt and Sylvia Lund and family; the Park Community Church family, and many friends.

Thank you for your love and care.

Tribute

An amazing person, Carol Ashwood, challenged me to reach new heights of living as she encouraged my writing and planted the thought of going to grad school. She has gently guided me through and beyond my darkest moments and never let go. It is because she continues to encourage me to view my life as worth living that I have learned what God's compassionate care and love are all about.

Thank you, Carol, for not giving up on me!

Contents

Introduction	1
Getting Affairs in Order	7
Diagnosis	13
The Stigma Remains	27
Elmer's Family	28
Adult Day Services	31
Support Group for Caregivers	32
Support Group Benefits	34
Medicare and Medicaid (Medical Assistance)	36
Overwhelmed Caregiver	39
Lack of Sleep	42
Growing Responsibilities	45
An Unwanted Role	48
Challenges	49
"Take Care of Yourself."—HOW?	51
Protecting the Image of My Loved One	54
Hypersexuality and Aggression	57
Help at Home Can Result in More Work for the Caregiver	61
Do You Think My Loved One Is Ready to Go to Memory Care?	65
Focus on the Caregiver's Well-Being	67
Focus on the Caregiver	68
Care Facilities and Memory Care Choices	71
Care Facilities	71
Memory Care	72
Placement in Memory Care	75
COVID-19	82

Guilt and Shame   85
- Unsuitable Coping Skills - Beer Bingeing and Suicidal Thoughts. 87
- Seeking Therapy 92
- Technology 96

Graduate School   101
- I Am Too Old 101

Hospice   105
- Hospice Again and Again. 106
- Hospice Facts and Who Qualifies 109
- Final Days of Life. 114

Widowhood   117
- Addictions and Suicides Among Older Widows and Widowers 119
- GriefShare: Grief is Not Something 'To Get Over' 123
- A Place at the Table (APATT) 125

I Have a Purpose   127

Resources   131
- Differences between Power of Attorney and Guardianship. 131
- Parts of An Elder Care Legal Plan 132
- Comparison of Elder Law Attorneys and Estate Attorneys 134
- Medical Terms 136
- A Successful Support Group 138
- Steps for Caregiver Support 139
- Memory Care Planning Assistance 141

References   143

About the Author   145

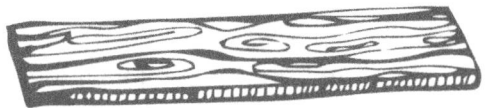

Introduction

Navigating the intricate path of dementia caregiving is like walking on a fog-shrouded bridge over troubled waters where we see only the deck and not the condition of the underside.

No one knows when a caregiver's bridge may collapse.

I gradually became the caregiver of my husband, Louis, as his diagnosis of depression worsened for twelve years before he was diagnosed with late-stage dementia caused by Alzheimer's disease. He went on to live another eight years, and during that time, I encountered insurmountable challenges. It did not get better once he was no longer at home, as bingeing on beer late into the evenings became my attempt to cope with the emotional pain, waves of shame, and the helplessness of not knowing whether Louis was in any pain—because he could not communicate.

My needs and those of my husband changed frequently as the disease progressed. I hid many struggles beneath the words, "I'm fine," because I did not want to disturb the busy lives of family and friends or have them think less of Louis. It was difficult to ask for help because I did not know what I needed, what was available, what was reasonable, and what was worth pursuing.

When the caregiver reaches a point where they can no longer provide adequate care for the individual at home, they are faced with the agonizing choice to move their loved one to a long-term care facility. To take Louis from our house to memory care was the most difficult decision on my journey, but I urgently needed to focus on my health and not the condition of my husband. I waited too long, anticipating that, as he was on the waiting list, it would only take a day or two to get him into a room. I was wrong! Something else I learned was that the burdens and challenges I faced did not simply disappear when Louis eventually left our home.

I have witnessed firsthand from three perspectives the physical and emotional toil of caring for a spouse with dementia:

- as the caregiver of my late husband with Alzheimer's disease
- as a Master of Science in Gerontology
- as a registered nurse (RN) in long-term care

Much strength is required to make it across the bridge of caregiving. The progression to death of a person with dementia can be very long, with little or no communication possible. This is unlike illnesses in which the caregiver has clear, meaningful interaction with the one they are caring for until their final days of life.

Though research acknowledges some challenges caregivers face, more is needed to understand and raise awareness of the journey from the caregiver's perspective. Many caregivers die within a couple of years before or after their spouse, and the increase in suicide rates among widows and widowers over the age of eighty is on the rise. Dementia significantly affects not only its sufferer and their spouse but also family and friends (Leggett et al. 2020). Bridges are collapsing.

For this reason, my primary goal is to share my own experience to help professionals, friends, and families care for the caregiver of a spouse with dementia. However, I hope this book will also help those of you who are or have been the primary caregiver of your spouse. When current and former caregivers share weaknesses, failures, and struggles, we can help those who follow us learn what is needed to keep their bridges safe.

This book sheds light on the concealed survival struggles of caregivers, similar to what lies beneath the deck of a wood bridge made with planks. These challenges erode the caregiver's strength, like the river current erodes the submerged cross-beams that steady the bridge and the gusset plates that keep the supports together. Just as these bear the weight of the entire structure, so caregivers carry their often sudden responsibilities, juggling care, household duties, and sometimes a job or career without adequate preparation.

The privacy of marriage and the vows I made when we were married caused me to hide difficult situations and keep on caring for Louis long after I should have admitted my limitations. My embarrassment and shame led to ineffective coping strategies.

A marriage can sustain and obscure these difficulties just as the deck hides the gusset plates holding the supports together and masks the erosion of rotting posts beneath the surface of the water.

How can we who have been and are caregivers help keep the bridges of other caregivers in good condition so they can make it across their collapsing bridge without falling off? I have become a bridge inspector because I know what it was like to cross my bridge, which was shaking and swaying as though it were about to throw me into the river below.

The reconstruction of this metaphorical bridge seeks to expose the hidden challenges of dementia caregiving and provide a sturdy and well-supported deck for caregivers. By doing so, we help them navigate the tumultuous river of dementia care with stability and reduced risk of danger.

These frequently hidden dangers can be extreme stress, a lack of preparation for the unwelcome role of a caregiver, and marriage itself. All these factors can, in turn, lead to hidden problematic coping mechanisms, which further undermine the strength and integrity of the bridge. Just as a bridge may collapse when the supports erode from the strong currents of the water or as the gussets fail, caregivers may even die without people to reinforce their support structures.

If you are the caregiver or asked by a caregiver when they should place their loved one in care, how can you stay neutral and yet help them make that decision when they are so focused on the care recipient? It was the hardest decision I had ever had to make. In this book, I will share with you why I waited too long.

If you are a caregiver to your spouse who has any form of dementia such as Alzheimer's, vascular dementia, Lewy body dementia, or frontotemporal dementia, rest assured you will find help in the following pages.

If you are a professional or friend helping keep caregivers safe, consider yourself a bridge inspector. Caregivers need you to

INTRODUCTION

assist them in finding help by repairing the bridge with new wood to make it safe for them to get to the riverbank on the other side. We are all unique individuals, as are those we care for. Your hand could be all a caregiver needs to reach dry land and attempt to move on without their spouse.

> "There are only four kinds of people in the world
> —those who have been caregivers,
> those who are currently caregivers,
> those who will be caregivers,
> and those who will need caregivers."
>
> Rosalyn Carter
> *Former First Lady of the United States*

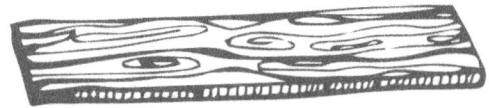

Getting Affairs in Order

My husband, Louis, had what seemed to be a transient ischemic attack (TIA) or mini-stroke. This is a temporary period of symptoms similar to those of a stroke—though, as some of the symptoms lingered on, Louis was later assumed rather to have had a seizure. I was confused as a neurologist advised me to get our affairs in order right away. My bewilderment was because, with only one child, it seemed clear our son was the beneficiary of everything we had. What else was there to do?

I was unaware of the additional legal documents needed for Louis' care. My only concern was having our assets, including our home, set up so that if something happened to both of us, our only child, Paul, would not have to deal with probate.

So I began to negotiate the perilous terrain of legal and medical jargon, a language that sounded foreign and confusing. What were the distinctions between Social Security, Medicare, Medicaid, Supplemental Security Income, Long Term Care Insurance, and, as we lived in Minnesota, Medical Assistance, Minnesota Care, and MN Sure? How did they connect to Medigap and Supplemental Health Insurance? Did I have to take the time to familiarize my already overloaded mind with those terms and how they applied to our circumstances? Why would I need Power of Attorney (POA) when I was his wife? What would it do? Was there a rush? What was a DPOA? What was guardianship? I learned we still needed a legal plan. The plan has five essential items and usually will eliminate dealing with probate, which is why you must have a revocable living trust as part of your estate plan. But then, what was the difference between an estate attorney and an elder law attorney?

I learned to interpret this convoluted language after realizing how crucial it was to planning our journey. It turned out that getting the Durable Power of Attorney (DPOA) was urgent. The rush was that my husband had to be able to understand and sign the legal DPOA documents and that they needed to be notarized in his presence.

Once I learned the importance of the DPOA, my husband, our son, and I met with an estate attorney, unaware that elder law attorneys specialize in addressing the needs and issues older citizens face. They are prepared to deal with concerns about healthcare, long-term care, government assistance, and prevention of elder abuse. While estate attorneys and elder law attorneys both deal with legal matters relating to people and their possessions, estate attorneys prepare documents for what to do with your possessions, including assets, *after you die*. I then discovered there was more legal jargon to quickly learn about trusts, living wills, wills, deeds, individual retirement accounts (IRAs), representative payees, guarantors, and so on.

It's essential to consult with an attorney specializing in elder law to assess your loved one's situation and determine the most appropriate, cost-effective, and timely course of action. They can provide guidance tailored to your jurisdiction's specific circumstances and legal requirements.

I learned that without the word 'durable', the power ends when a person becomes incapacitated, and the person they named in the document has no authority to help them. This includes a spouse or other family member, such as an adult child. We also created a DPOA for me, should our son ever need it. If there is no DPOA, guardianship may become the only option.

Ultimately, the choice between a DPOA and guardianship depends on the specific circumstances and the needs of the individual involved. If the person is still mentally competent and able to make decisions, establishing a DPOA is usually the best, least time-consuming, and least costly option. However, if someone has already lost decision-making capacity, guardianship may be necessary to protect their interests, even though it may be more expensive and involve court oversight.

The cost of setting up a DPOA versus obtaining guardianship can vary significantly based on several factors, including your location, the complexity of the situation, and the specific legal services required.

Selecting a 'package' from an attorney to get our affairs in order seemed expensive, but it needed to be done as soon as possible. When it was finished, I felt it had been well worth the cost. Since we only had one child, we had not considered setting up a living trust or will. Because we were a married couple and could protect each other, Louis and I had assumed there was no need for other legal documents.

Our son and I also had a vital meeting with a financial planner to decide how to manage the finances. It was a great relief for both him and me to have the DPOAs of finances and health care (also known as MN Health Care Directives) in place and to know everything was in order. Now, our son was also listed as a beneficiary of all our assets that required one. We learned that had we put the DPOA off any longer, we would have had to obtain the costly and more complex guardianship.

I used Louis' DPOA documents several times in the following eight years, keeping one in my car at all times and one in a safe. Our attorney also provided a computer zip drive, which made it easy to search for things.

There are many legal and medical terms involved in advocating more effectively for a spouse with dementia, making educated choices, and navigating the legal and healthcare systems successfully. Even though I was a registered nurse, the medical terminology and acronyms were overwhelming; it was like learning a new language without time to understand it fully. During my years of nursing, facilities with memory care were unheard of.

If you're in Minnesota, you can get free advice from a local 'aging expert' at the Senior LinkAge Line at 1-800-333-2433. This helps older adults and their families find community services or plan their future, and other states have similar resources.

I needed insights to prepare for our future. There were excellent community education workshops and much to learn while caring for Louis. Attending free seminars by elder law attorneys was very helpful. Often, the workshops offer a free consultation to determine current needs. Most will not pressure anyone to use their services, but they may also provide discounts if you do. You don't always need a lawyer to answer questions that come up later, and attorney offices usually have other staff who can help you.

All these things should be done long before signs of an upcoming crisis. I feel strongly that this information should be available in an information booklet—for older people, in particular, to consult long before any dementia diagnosis.

Under Resources at the back of this book, you will find a brief overview of the differences between power of attorney and guardianship, a comparison of elder law attorneys and estate attorneys, and the key components of an elder care legal plan.

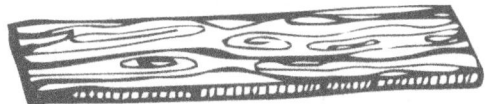

Diagnosis

The beginning of our fifty-three years of marriage was like stability on solid ground. Life was gentle, and the winds were calm. My husband was a man with no significant health issues and a wonderful father to our son.

Louis did not tell me when his primary physician diagnosed him with depression; he just mentioned high blood pressure. Whenever he went to his doctor, he would give me a brief report on medication to keep him stable. He never mentioned what can be an early indicator of dementia—depression.

The extremely gradual progression of Louis' depression was complex and began about twenty years before he died. I initially mistook subtle cognitive changes as signs of depression rather than dementia, attributing it to the death of his mother, new ownership at his work, the loss of his job, and rotator cuff surgery he had been putting off for a couple of years. In hindsight, for over a dozen years, I overlooked the early red flags, as did his primary physician. Despite there being no improvement in his depression, it took over twelve years until he was given the diagnosis of late-stage dementia caused by Alzheimer's disease.

There were gradual changes as Louis struggled to work with numbers. He dodged several things, like figuring out tips when we were eating out. One difference I missed was when a couple of best friends used to go out for lunch with us on Sundays after church. Louis began to look at how much of a tip they gave and put down the same amount for us. A few years later, he asked me to use my credit card, reasoning that I could get it out more easily. It seemed sensible, and I did not notice him losing his ability to use numbers. I now understand how easy it is to attribute early symptoms of dementia, like working with numbers, to other causes. I thought people with dementia got lost or forgot the names of family members, but Louis was not living in the past like that.

He was spending more time at work and coming home later and later. Urgent projects took more time and planning before he even started them, and he would begin projects but not finish them. I thought nothing of this as his workload seemed to increase, and I knew Louis was a well-liked people pleaser. Without thinking, I began to help him more with little things.

I didn't detect any cause for alarm in these little ripples, and we had been married for over thirty years when they became more like waves.

His workplace was somewhere Louis loved to be. He rarely complained about work, and when a printing press broke down, he would stay extra hours and learn from the specialized press mechanics. He delighted in understanding new things and cared for the building and equipment as if he owned them.

He was working longer and longer on numerous projects. He would call to let me know he'd be at work for another couple of hours. I often took him a late evening meal and stayed up to four hours to help him. Often, we worked together on projects. I am grateful for all that I learned and the opportunity to assist. We were a couple and cared for each other as husband and wife usually do.

Louis was a handyman with lots of skills, and he was also a workaholic, but now, I can look back and see more clearly some of the symptoms that were the beginning of dementia.

Our life continued as usual until Louis was released from the job he had held and loved for forty-two years. He had begun as a pressman with five other employees, and all those years later, there were over forty. Louis was only sixty-one and devastated. The new company owners appeared to be struggling financially, so it made some sense to him that he was let go. Later, I discovered he had become overwhelmed by his projects as building superintendent. His enthusiasm for going to work each day had been very slowly declining. With no chance of returning, my husband was given some severance pay and three months to empty his office and retrieve his tools.

Louis then studied to become a school bus driver but lost the confidence to pass the written test before taking it. This difficulty was one of my earliest concerns that he was losing some critical cognitive abilities. He kept busy with his volunteer responsibilities at our church, including managing the heating plant. A few years later, when our water heater failed, Louis did not feel confident replacing it, which was unusual. The other cognitive changes over the next four years were not very noticeable, except that he slept more during the day and seemed more depressed.

I waited for several years for Louis to get some bids for new siding on our house and finally realized he could no longer make comparisons or figure out whom to call. I carefully asked if it was okay for me to go ahead and see what we could get, expecting him to want to put it off another year. In previous years, when I'd suggested it, he would dismiss it with, "I think it can wait a year." Instead, he responded with a sigh of relief and suggested we have the windows replaced simultaneously. I had not thought about the old windows, so I took his good advice and went ahead and found a contractor.

Louis now looked to me for all decisions and agreed with whatever I said. Making home maintenance decisions independently when he was still with me at home seemed awkward, yet I learned those responsibilities were now solely resting on me. I was handling all the finances and also maintaining our home, our cabin until it was sold, and our two vehicles.

When I came home from work one day, I was greeted by an apprehensive whimpering dog, who led me to find my husband curled up in a fetal position on the floor, sound asleep. I woke him to find his speech slurred and confused, though he had good vital signs and no obvious weakness. We headed to an emergency room where a battery of tests were done, including Magnetic Resonance Imaging (MRI), with no definite diagnosis. He was put on hospital observation with apparent mini-seizures or mini-strokes. Over four days, his speech improved, though he still found numbers, dates, and times to be stumbling blocks.

I later learned that hospital 'observation' meant Medicare would not cover him for the first twenty days of direct admission to a licensed care facility such as a hospital or nursing home. A patient had to be 'admitted' for a minimum of three days for Medicare to cover the first twenty days, and the next eighty days was a co-pay only if the person was discharged from a hospital after being admitted and had been there for at least those three days. After that, being at a licensed care facility would require private pay from any assets we had. Licensed care facilities may include hospitals, nursing homes, memory care units, hospice care facilities, and some assisted living. It's important to note that state licensing varies.

Louis was thought to be having subclinical seizures that had been going on for some time—perhaps several years. He did fine with regular conversations, but comprehension was a problem. Sometimes, he would repeat questions. If asked to do something with more than one step to it, he hesitated in starting on it.

The neurologist felt a need to prevent any more seizures from occurring by placing Louis on a preventative seizure drug and prescribing occupational therapy to help regain some of the skills he had lost. The medication was very sedative, causing him to sleep much of the daytime.

Louis could not do a simple addition of two single numbers. He asked for a calculator to add four plus three. After three sessions of six appointments for occupational therapy, the therapist advised the neurologist that Louis was not getting better and told us to make an appointment as soon as possible with a different neurologist for a second opinion. The 'as soon as possible' meant a wait of four months.

I had heard lots of things about Alzheimer's, but each person is unique. Though his cognitive impairment deteriorated rapidly over the next two years, Louis still knew where he was, that his parents had died, and where they were buried, and he recognized people by name. I found it hard to make any comparisons to others with dementia. Many books only seemed to cover things like how to respond when people with dementia have forgotten a family member has died and how not to make them deal with the loss all over again.

Over the following two years, we tried to get appointments with the neurologist, who would simply make tiny changes in Louis' meds and tell us to come back in two weeks. This was a test of my patience as two weeks, no matter how I insisted, always ended up being five to six months. With the current shortages in medical staffing, these long waits will only get longer, and new patients may need to wait a year for an appointment. This is when I started to feel flooded by medical terminology that even I, a registered nurse, didn't recognize.

Louis rapidly lost his confidence in driving and depended on me to do all of it. He often waited for me to get home and then asked me to drive him places in his truck. It was good that I did like to drive because now, on long drives to our cabin, he slept. His truck was also his tool shed on wheels, but I found it hard to switch roles and be the one asking for specific tools from the truck. He was always happy to help, though.

I needed to be reminded that Louis was still capable of helping me even after he was diagnosed with Alzheimer's disease. If he could not do a task one day, I lacked the patience to wait another day or even another hour for him maybe to figure it out. I sensed Louis' trust in my ability to use power tools and tried not to act surprised that he had lost his confidence in them. It was important to be aware of what he did have confidence in using, and he kept much of his understanding of safety with tools while he remained at home.

There were moments of guilt when I didn't allow enough time for Louis to get dressed or failed to put his clothes out in an orderly manner. He continued to enjoy our church work day as long as I stayed in sight nearby. The guys were great at finding things for him to do and keeping an eye on him, but Louis wanted to be able to see me. Once, I noticed that his jeans were starting to fall off. How could that be? Before we left the house, I had checked to see that his belt was on. However, it turned out there was more to check on because jeans without a belt actually threaded through the loops tend to gravitate to the ground. Fortunately, a friend of Lou's offered to fix what could have been an embarrassing disaster. In moments like this, it felt respectful that no attention was drawn to my error as the caregiver or to Louis' problems, like keeping his pants up.

When you are around someone with dementia, if there is an opportunity to help, offer to do so or simply silently help if you know the family well. Remind yourself that you have no idea what the caregiver has already dealt with that day.

I put our lake cabin on the market as Louis could no longer help me with the upkeep. We rarely spent time there since it was two hundred miles away, and there was no purpose in keeping it up when we no longer used it. I was grateful for my farm upbringing because closing up the cabin for winter each year involved crawling into a lengthy crawl space, disposing of dead critters, and draining water lines and the water heater. It was something Louis could no longer do, nor was he worried that I wouldn't get it right. It was a year of many changes for me amid the growing dementia issues of my husband.

That fall, we did our usual volunteer work at the Lake Region Pioneer Threshermen's Show in Dalton, MN, including the prep work to clean and ready the print shop there that Louis had been supervising for several years. Louis did make it clear to the shop crew and me that he would no longer run the old letterpress or cutter. Instead, he kept everything clean, sat outside at the door most of the time, and opened and locked up each night.

He had taught me about preserving the equipment for the winter and the many months when it was idle, such as using bed sheets for covers from the dust and not plastic tarps, as steel needs to breathe. A month later, he reminded me that we had not done that when we cleaned up. As we put bed sheets over the equipment later that fall, Louis sadly told me he thought he could not manage the shop any longer. I offered to be with him the following year, which made him very happy! The smile on his face was a rare delight.

The next year, when we went to clean before the three-day show, he just watched me. He was puzzled when I gave him a broom to sweep the floor, though he figured it out when I handed him the dustpan. On the show's second day, Daryl, a friend from our church in the Twin Cities, came unannounced and asked Louis to show him the threshing grounds while I worked in the print shop. Those five hours were the longest time for over a year that he hadn't needed me to be in his sight every moment. I had forgotten what it was like to feel such freedom, and it was a surprise gift from Daryl I will never forget.

At home, Louis had become touchier. He would admit he could not figure something out and would get frustrated, asking me for help. When I tried to help him, he would say, "If you know so much about it, then do it!" or, "Why can't you help?" It made no difference whether I helped or not; he would get upset with me. It was another test of my patience!

After five minutes of weed trimming, Louis would be exhausted and have to stop. It took him three hours to do what he had done the previous year in an hour. One day, he was cleaning the lawn mower air filter. As he finished, he asked me if he should pour gas or clean oil on the filter before putting it back on the engine. Putting gas on it could have resulted in a fire the next time it was started, and it was a good reminder that I needed to be at his side whenever he worked with tools or tried to clean or fix anything. My stress was increasing as I watched him and attempted to figure out whether he was doing something correctly or if I dared to offer help. At times, I would sneak back and redo what he had done to keep his pride in being able to do things.

Louis lost confidence in doing anything while I was at work. He slept in front of the TV, and there were days when he didn't touch the lunch I had set out for him. He would be hungry when I came home, asking how long before supper.

He got more depressed and frustrated with himself, saying, "I can't do anything right anymore!" and, "I can't do anything!" In public, he didn't talk much to anyone. He no longer answered the phone unless he thought it was me, and it often took a couple of calls in a row for him to figure out how to answer it.

From being a skilled handyman, Louis became increasingly incapable within a year. He struggled to operate the washing machine and would rely on me to mow the lawn. His memory and problem-solving skills gradually declined, and he avoided tasks that had become difficult. He panicked when unable to find or understand something, such as the purpose of the pull cord on the snow blower. My questions got one-word responses of "Okay" and "Fine." However, he still excelled at recognizing people.

After more cognitive decline, we sought a second opinion about Louis' diagnosis of seizures, this time from a neurologist specializing in epilepsy, known as an epileptologist. She suspected he had not had any seizures but rather a TIA, or mini-stroke, as there was no weakness and had only been a few hours of slurred speech and confusion. Abby, our dog, was the only witness to whatever happened before I came home and found him tightly curled up on the floor that day.

I could not imagine Abby being helpful in a diagnosis; however, one unusual question the epileptologist had was about the dog's reaction when I came into the house that day. She was whimpering and led me straight to Louis and lay down tightly next to him. Abby had not been afraid, as some dogs are after witnessing a grand mal seizure.

There was brain atrophy present in Louis' MRI from two years before, meaning that some dementia was present even before that time. This new doctor affirmed that numerous little TIAs instead of subclinical seizures may have been occurring but that the ups and downs were more typical of dementia.

Within four weeks of first visiting the epileptologist, she changed the initial diagnosis of depression to late-stage Alzheimer's disease, which causes progressive dementia. Louis was sent the following week to the University of Minnesota Memory Care Clinic next door for confirmation of the diagnosis. The doctor there confirmed the diagnosis and told us to return in a couple of weeks for a family meeting. Louis' Alzheimer's disease was much more advanced than I expected.

An early diagnosis is difficult. However, many other conditions that are treatable share symptoms with dementia—conditions such as vitamin deficiencies, thyroid dysfunction, urinary tract infection, alcohol abuse, dehydration, blood clots, brain tumors, head injuries, side effects of medication, kidney or liver problems, anxiety, stress, and depression.

The immediate impression one gets after a diagnosis of dementia is that the individual has been written off as one who, in a day, has become worthless to society. In our case, Louis' world changed to one of shame and despair. Trying to encourage him when no one else did was hard. I was also losing some sense of my safety as his wife due to his unusual agitation at home.

Not having a diagnosis for so long had kept the stigma of Alzheimer's away for a while, for which I am grateful. Instead of discussing concerns and asking for assistance, I had chosen to surround my husband in an environment of normalization to protect and preserve his independence and dignity. Due to the stigma we as a couple dealt with afterward, I would not have wanted to hear the diagnosis of disease-causing progressive dementia any earlier than we did. To have several years without it provided us with more everyday living.

When using the three stages of dementia as the early stage, the mid-stage, and the final or end stage, Louis was already past the mid-stage and in the final stage, struggling with more noticeable progression of the disease. Research on medications to slow it down provides no proof that any drug is effective in stopping the progression, eliminating dementia, or making it better. You will find more extensive information in an excellent free webinar, "A New Era: Understanding Lecanemab, Donanemab, and Emerging Therapies for Alzheimer's Disease." It is directed by Dr. Joseph E. Gaugler of the University of Minnesota School of Public Health and was presented on November 6, 2023. It's available at https://youtu.be/DUtQq9Aa3WU.

Louis' diagnosis had a significant impact on my life, as my future immediately changed. He seemed to understand and was silent until we got home, but the diagnosis was jarring, and it was one of the very few times he ever cried. He never mentioned anything about his diagnosis after that day but became relatively silent.

However, Louis was now very aware of struggling with numbers and time. He felt ashamed when, during med-check appointments, he could not draw a clock or figure out where to put the numbers. When we came home from the five-minute meeting in which he was asked by a physician's assistant (PA) to remember three objects, he would be very upset with me for not helping him when I was at his side in the clinic office. I emailed the PA, who assured Louis that he would never again be asked to draw a clock or remember three objects. That was the end of individual appointments while he was living at home.

The most challenging part of the diagnosis was that Louis could no longer be left alone. "Get your affairs in order; I don't need to see you again," is often how a doctor ends a dementia diagnosis. I needed to know as soon as possible what to do, but the clinics provided no practical guidance on what to expect or where to turn for help, no encouragement, no hope, and no information about how to live with this complex condition. I did not know there were adult day services in our area or internet sites like alzheimers.gov, which you will find at https://www.alzheimers.gov/life-with-dementia/tips-caregivers.

On top of the list of shocking things to find out was that having Medicare and a good health insurance supplement would not cover the cost when Louis might need care in a licensed facility such as a nursing home or memory care.

Even if I anticipated the diagnosis, like all caregivers, I needed help adjusting to this new reality. I still had a full-time job. I did not know what to do about leaving Louis home alone, as he seemed to sleep most of the time while 'watching' television and was not incontinent. A week later, I found out that instead of looking for an adult babysitter, I should be looking for adult day services. I saw a brochure about some kind of walk to end Alzheimer's, which I ignored as I thought the Alzheimer's Association at alz.org was only for raising money for a cure and wouldn't have help or information for caregivers. Later, I learned about support groups they sponsored and joined one that provided incredible help with caregiving and knowing I was not alone.

I was told that a social worker and a neurologist would see us for an hour at a family meeting "in a couple of weeks." There was no information about what a family meeting was, who should come, or any other information that would have been so helpful, and it took five months to get an appointment. The family meeting was worthless; we were just asked if we had any questions, but I didn't know what I needed or what was available that I might find helpful. By then, it was too late for questions, anyway, as it was when Louis was diagnosed five months earlier that I needed to know about day services available, among many other things. It was also dehumanizing to have a new doctor talking to us as if Louis wasn't there or couldn't understand anything the doctor said. The social worker was silent and had no information for us. That scheduled hour-long meeting lasted twenty minutes.

Lack of assistance for the caregiver following a diagnosis contributes to the misconception that people living with dementia have no options. If we are to persuade people to seek care for a dementia diagnosis, the norm must include positive representations of people living well with dementia and receiving support to maintain their independence and autonomy. This, rather than the catastrophic perspectives sometimes shown in the media.

The river of dementia is unforgiving, and the bridge I had to use to cross it confronted me with challenges that felt impassable. This is a river that reveals the accurate measure of one's character and the strength of the bonds we share with our loved ones. A deep heartache I had to face was that I could do nothing to fix things as intimate communication with my husband slowly drifted away.

Under Resources, you will find a short list of medical terms that might be helpful.

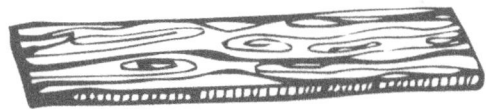

The Stigma Remains

The stigma of dementia has not ended. However, there have been changes in care as more is learned about over 125 progressive diseases that cause it.

In the 1800s and early 1900s, horror stories were spread of families who sent loved ones to the 'lunatic asylums' (state hospitals) when they could no longer care for them at home. Relatives were often ashamed of their loved one's behavior and said very little. They were also afraid that their loved ones might tell negative, untrue stories and that those listening would believe them.

Restraints were gradually replaced with sedatives and antipsychotics, and most state hospitals have closed. From the 1950s, many residents of those hospitals ended up in nursing homes, but it took years before the Internet in 1983 and the World Wide Web in 1993 could spread the word about improvements in caregiving. Since then, medical communication has seen remarkable changes, including information on how to care for people with dementia.

Elmer's Family

In the 1970s and 1980s, I worked as a night supervisor in a 213-bed suburban nursing home. At night, the dementia patients were often restrained to protect them from wandering and falls.

I remember well a little man whom I'll call Elmer. Even when we took away his clock, he got up every morning at 4:30 a.m. and tried to get out of the nursing home. Our staff continued to catch him, return him to his bed, and sometimes restrain him, as he would be combative about insisting he had to get out, though he never said why. One busy early morning, Elmer evaded other staff and, in -20°F weather, headed out the front door with his jacket over his pajamas. I prepared for a freezing outdoor chase. To my surprise, I found Elmer sitting on a bench outside the door. After pumping his fists for half a minute, he returned, seeming very satisfied, and went back to bed.

The following morning, I watched Elmer go outside to see if he would again sit on the bench and return within a minute. He did! I realized Elmer had been a farmer and asked him if he was tending to his farm work. He said, "The cows always have to be milked," and returned to his bed.

I was still concerned because it was frigid outside. The next night, I set the little bench he sat on between the sets of double doors in the entry so he would not be exposed to the cold air. Early that morning, Elmer went out to the bench and cared for his cows. On returning to bed, I asked him how the milking went. "Well, it was much better today because I finally got the ice chipped out so I could close the north barn door." How much more manageable and satisfying it was for our staff to move the bench each morning instead of restraining him. I now had a satisfied farmer, not an unruly patient.

Elmer taught me so much when I took the time and patience to allow him to share with me his family of seven cows. Like my dad's, every cow had a name, and Elmer never forgot their names or the order in which he milked them. I heard delightful early morning stories about each cow and how she acquired her name. When his physical health made it impossible for Elmer to care for his cows, our staff offered to take care of them and report back to him. One morning, he said, "Can you believe it? Marge even cleaned my barn!"

Every person with Alzheimer's is different, and we now know more about dementia care because so much has been shared. Caregivers learn to respond to their loved ones and others according to the moment they're in rather than trying to correct them. There are special moments we can share with folks like Elmer, who had no human family but was devoted to his unique family of cows.

However, though medical communication has seen remarkable changes in how we care for people with dementia, the stigma remains.

Very few people want to go to a nursing home or a memory care facility, and few desire to work in one. What reasonable changes are possible as nursing homes close due to a lack of both staff and funds? Simply raising wages does no good if there is no one to pay. Now is the time for us all to think of how we can influence our future, design an environment that needs fewer medical professionals, and make their work more enjoyable. If workers don't know they are part of saving lives, how can we communicate to them their importance?

Caregivers need those who stand by and step in to help. However, though the outward appearance of my husband did not change overnight the day he was diagnosed, there was a noticeable change in how we were treated by others. For many of our friends, awareness of Louis' diagnosis seemed to trigger immediate discomfort. We received the silent treatment as though we suddenly had a contagious disease. When we were around groups of people, they seemed to avoid us. This sudden shift in behavior from warm and friendly to distant and aloof was a stark reminder of the profound misconceptions surrounding dementia. He was treated as though he was suddenly incapable of doing what he had been able to do a day or week before. There had been no blunt force trauma. Louis could still walk. He could still hang up his coat on a hanger. He could still use the restroom.

I now felt expected to be at Louis' side every moment. In public, he was fine going to the restroom by himself, but as early as the week following the dementia diagnosis, friends expected me to go with him. Sitting around tables for coffee with church friends, where I sat with a table of women and Louis with a table of men, now seemed unacceptable. Even when there was no room, people would add a chair for us to sit together, but I longed for those coffee times just to have some separation.

Louis was not one to respond inappropriately to people, and though he became very quiet, he continued to know who people were and enjoyed listening to conversations. He seemed to be at his best whenever other people were near. At home with me, he was very different, and both of us felt the isolation as Louis grappled with the shame of his condition. Navigating these challenges of caregiving served to increase my emotional exhaustion. We were shouldering the burden of not just the disease itself but also the stigma that surrounded it.

The stigma of Alzheimer's disease does not discriminate; it impacts not only the person diagnosed but also their caregivers and family. It was very encouraging to read in the "Alzheimer's Spouse Journal and Support Group" on Facebook that I was not alone.

Dementia brought some dramatic changes. One of the most heart-wrenching aspects was witnessing Louis's anxiety when I was out of his sight. I couldn't hide, nor did I want to. It was saddening to see him so desperately cling to the sight of me, his eyes reflecting the deep fear of losing track of me. He became determined to keep me in his sight at all times, whether we were home or away. Eventually, I removed the bathroom door in case he had a seizure and I needed to get in, but he did not notice it was gone. It was all a stark reminder of the extent to which dementia had reshaped our lives.

The weight of Louis' well-being and mine rested squarely on my shoulders. The responsibility to protect him became an ever-present burden as he increasingly relied on me for assistance. The toll was unrelenting. No private moments were left for me—no peaceful showers, no shopping alone, and no nights of restful sleep. It was as though every second of my day was devoted to his care.

Adult Day Services

When my husband could no longer be at home alone, I felt guilty for deciding to place him in adult day services at a place called the Colonial Club so I could continue to work at my full-time job. Louis still valued that I was bringing in an income, and he rode with me to work so I could drop him off for his morning coffee at the 'Club'. A bus from the facility brought him back about an hour before I got home. He would doze in his recliner, often unaware of when I returned.

I could not imagine my caregiving stress could increase any further. However, as Louis' condition worsened, I received a notice that the Colonial Club was closing. It was more to deal with, but in the end, it was also a blessing. A different facility for adult day services with longer hours, DayBridge, allowed me to drop Louis off on my way to work and pick him up on my way home. He was not excited to attend, but he didn't complain. At the end of each day, he anxiously waited at the door for me, and his silent displeasure was heartbreaking.

Support Group for Caregivers

I noticed a community education booklet listing a support group for the carers of people with Alzheimer's and other dementia. The twice-a-month meetings with an experienced facilitator were the most incredible support in steadying my bridge. It was similar to having a bridge inspector who finds repairs that are needed and writes a work order. However, a support group is not just for dealing with your challenges but for being able to share what may be helpful to others. Group members responded to questions and shared difficulties.

The facilitator recognized how vital it was to assist one another and encouraged us to share how we had handled a specific challenge, emphasizing that no two people are alike. To assist us, she followed up with precise, often printed information whenever she could. She made it 'our time' to know we were not only there for help but also had a purpose—helping others. When anyone made a suggestion, they were asked if they had tried it and if it had succeeded. We would have two weeks to give it a go or explain why we hadn't. When something did not work, we learned from others what else they had tried and what might be effective in our situations. A truth I heard from other caregivers was, "It only gets worse." Their honesty humbled me!

Finding a support group that suits your needs and preferences is essential. Some support groups meet in person, while others may convene online, offering flexibility suited to your schedule and comfort level. Additionally, they may focus on specific aspects of caregiving or cater to different types of dementia, so choose one that aligns with your situation if possible.

Support groups should be spaces where you can share and support one another without having to listen to a speaker. I did not need to hear about how a diagnosis was obtained when I already knew. For example, I wanted to learn how others were finding help with keeping their spouses active.

It became very important to me to regularly attend a group that meets twice a month. It felt essential to meet more than monthly as caregiving challenges escalate frequently. We met in person before COVID-19, and then during the shutdown, we met remotely on Zoom. This meant the meeting did not have to be close by, and caregivers didn't have to find someone to be with their loved ones while attending. COVID-19 pushed the use of technology and eliminated the need to drive to a meeting.

Our group usually had a three-minute introduction by the facilitator. Then, time to speak was divided equally among those present, ensuring all had the option to share or pass. Time management is essential in facilitating discussion for those who may be shy and would be left out by dominant attendees who might not keep track of time. Support groups remind us that we are not alone, and it is not okay for someone needing support to wait another two weeks or a month to get help simply because time is poorly managed. However, time and keeping responses to a minimum with different people sharing can be among the most challenging things to control.

Support Group Benefits

- **Emotional Support:** Caregiving for a spouse with dementia can be emotionally challenging. Support groups provide a safe space to express your feelings, fears, and frustrations. Sharing your experiences with others who understand can be cathartic and reduce feelings of isolation.

- **Information and Education:** Support group facilitators may provide educational materials to help caregivers better understand dementia, its progression, and how to manage common caregiving challenges. Time is valuable and should be divided equally as much as possible between attendees rather than having a speaker take away time from them, as topics do not apply to all. It is invaluable to share personal struggles and accomplishments with those who have some understanding and compassion.

- **Practical Advice:** Caregivers can exchange helpful tips and strategies for managing daily tasks, communicating with their spouse, and handling behavioral changes often accompanying dementia. Keeping up with technology is always a challenge. A Jiobit on a shoelace tracks a wandering person with your cell phone's GPS and works inside most shopping malls. An alarm attached to the back of a garment alerts the caregiver when a loved one tries to get out of bed or a chair.

- **Reducing Stress:** Caregiving can be physically and mentally exhausting. Support groups can offer stress management techniques and coping strategies to help caregivers better manage their well-being.
- **Peer Perspective:** Hearing about the experiences and solutions of other caregivers can provide valuable insights and help you see you are not alone in facing the challenges of caregiving.
- **Social Interaction:** Caregiving can be isolating, and support groups allow social interaction and connection with others who share similar experiences. Building friendships within the group can reduce feelings of loneliness.
- **Problem-Solving:** Group members often brainstorm solutions to common caregiving problems, providing innovative approaches to challenging situations as well as practical advice. For example, the electronic medication dispensers seem to be fail-proof as they beep when it is time to take medication and allow a person to remove only that dose. However, the person may dispose of a tablet rather than swallowing it.
- **Respite Care Information:** Support groups can provide information on respite care options, allowing caregivers to take much-needed breaks to rest and recharge.
- **Advocacy and Resources:** Some support groups may offer information about local resources, legal and financial guidance, and advocacy efforts related to dementia care.
- **Validation:** Sharing your experiences and challenges with others can validate your feelings and experiences, helping you realize that your struggles are real and justified.

Under Resources, you will find more information about what makes a successful support group.

Medicare and Medicaid (Medical Assistance)

One caregiver may have a tightly-knit support network, while another might face the challenge of caregiving alone. Finances are pivotal in caregiving, whether navigating the complexities of government assistance, managing a substantial inheritance, or coping with private pay. Mistakes can be significant and life-altering. In Minnesota, the surviving spouse does not need to move out of their home to pay for the care of a spouse in a nursing home who qualifies for Medicaid (medical assistance). However, assets such as life insurance policies with cash values must be used. Many states put a lien against the home of a married couple so the spouse at home, who may be referred to as the community spouse, has a place to live the rest of their life.

For many, rehabilitation after an injury or illness is their first introduction to long-term care. Though these rehabilitation stints are often short-term, the admission process is similar to the application process for permanent placement in a nursing home.

While federally-run Medicare does cover the costs of skilled nursing rehabilitation for a few days, there are limitations. Remember, Medicare coverage today kicks in only if the patient has been previously admitted to a hospital for at least three days—rather than merely kept under observation—with a plan for safe discharge from the hospital to a licensed skilled facility. And while Medicare Part A provides limited inpatient rehabilitation coverage, this is capped at one hundred days. Complete coverage of licensed rehabilitation facility costs is provided only during the first twenty days, with copayments applicable for days twenty-one to one hundred. So, while

Medicare covers most of the costs of a typical rehabilitation stay—usually limited to a non-private room—after a hundred days, there is no coverage. Health insurance does not cover long-term care, memory care, or assisted living care.

The American Council on Aging provides current information on eligibility for Medicaid in each state and helps with the qualifying process. They offer a free, fast, non-binding Medicaid long-term care eligibility test, which you can find at https://www.medicaidplanningassistance.org/medicaid-eligibility-test/.

For the section, "Answers to All of Your Questions About Medicaid Long Term Care," see their FAQs at: https://www.medicaidplanningassistance.org/medicaid-long-term-care-faq/.

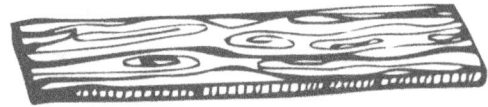

Overwhelmed Caregiver

Caring for a partner with a debilitating condition such as dementia is a profoundly challenging and emotionally charged journey. This caregiving role often takes a heavy toll on the caregivers, manifesting in a decline in their physical and emotional stamina. The complexities of this experience and its emotional and psychological aspects cannot be underestimated. The intense emotional demands of caregiving, coupled with changes in the intimacy of marriage due to dementia, can also amplify existing emotional vulnerabilities.

Caring for my husband before my retirement was not my plan; I had lost my passion for direct patient care in nursing and changed careers, and I was now working full-time as an office manager. Yet, the demands of caregiving increased.

I grappled with the emotional turmoil of witnessing the gradual erosion of Louis' capabilities, all the while striving to provide the best care possible. Though tested by uncertainty and grief, my love remained a beacon of hope and unwavering support.

People were telling me how they expected me to live. A relative heard the diagnosis of Alzheimer's and immediately responded, "It's good you're a nurse, so you can retire and care for him at home." My anger in those moments had a very narrow focus: I wanted to lash back because of how the words hurt. I knew I did not have the patience to care for Lou at home forever. Today, I might not be silent, but at the time, I was at a very low point, even thinking of ways to end my life.

There were gradual changes to adjust to in Louis' condition as I searched for all the information I could find, but as his wife, it was difficult to notice many of them. I felt helpless, not knowing what I needed. Taking Louis grocery shopping with me and getting him to hold onto a cart was very time-consuming. Once, I thought he was following me with the cart, but he was suddenly not in sight. At least I knew he was not ahead of me, but my retreat to the previous aisle found him, not the cart. I also had to apologize to other shoppers a few times because Louis had switched carts. He was unhappy that I was giving "our cart" to someone else.

Lawn mowing was a task we had shared that now became mine. Before he sat outside to watch me, I would have him pull the starter cord so he would feel needed. One day, he came to me wanting to help mow, so I let him. He forgot about holding the mower handle for it to run until I explained why it was shutting off. Focusing on holding the handle was the limit of his thinking, and he broke into a sweat while I mustered the patience not to try to correct him. After only a few minutes, he wore out and was glad when I relieved him. He had mowed repeatedly in a small circle, but it was great to see the smiling satisfaction on his face at being able to help.

There were all kinds of possible solutions for the problems that came up, but some of my attempts were a disaster. It was not like negotiating with an aging parent with dementia; we had been married for a long time, and Louis followed every step I took, even in the house. Even our bathroom was no longer a room of privacy.

Louis's sister occasionally came to help. She took long weekends off work and took him out to visit relatives while he still recognized them. When his driver's license needed renewal, she offered to take him one day to get an ID card in its place. It was a relief to let her take care of it.

Louis had no desire for a license; his pickup was sitting in our driveway because he no longer had confidence in his driving. I needed to keep the battery from dying during the winter, and Louis had a boiler operator's license and managed the heating system at our church. Making this a routine every Saturday kept the truck going, and Louis felt useful on weekends as we checked that all heating systems were running fine. He would eagerly brush off any snow beforehand so the truck was ready for me to drive.

I did not have it in my heart to sell the truck, as he still wanted me to drive it every time we ventured out together. It was also his tool shed on wheels. He was unaware I had switched the ignition key on his keychain to an old one, knowing that men with keys in pockets are like women with purses. I was concerned he might forget he did not have a license and try to drive. On the battery, I put a note with my phone number to call before attempting to jump-start it, as I worried he might try to put a charger on it. Whether Louis could dial my number was questionable, but if something happened to me, a serviceman would also see the note.

The caregiving journey is exhaustive, demanding tremendous physical and emotional energy. From assisting with daily activities to managing medical appointments and constantly adapting to the evolving needs of a partner with dementia, I found myself stretched to my limits. I have experienced how this relentless cycle can lead to physical exhaustion, sleep disturbances, and even chronic health issues from the wear and tear that comes with providing round-the-clock care.

Lack of Sleep

The challenges seemed insurmountable, and I yearned for even a single night of uninterrupted sleep. The relentless exhaustion stemmed from a ritual that spanned two agonizing years. I kept an ear out after each of the half dozen or more trips Louis made to the bathroom from 11 p.m. to at least 3 a.m. His anxiety may have been about bedwetting, something that never transpired.

In the cruel grip of dementia, he would forget within moments that he had just been to the bathroom, and every night, the cycle would repeat itself for those three to four hours. The difficult aspect of this nightly ordeal, and why it kept me awake, was that Louis left the bathroom sink water running each time. It didn't matter how often I gently reminded him to turn off the water, how clearly I articulated my request, or even if I left a note on the bathroom mirror as a visual cue. My reminders made no difference. His inability to grasp this simple task was emblematic of the unrelenting progression of dementia, a cruel thief that rapidly stole not only his cognitive abilities but also my sleep.

I learned from other caregivers to focus on the brighter moments. Most nights, keeping a light on at his bedside and in the bathroom kept Louis from wandering downstairs, but one night at 3 a.m., I heard my husband in the kitchen happily putting away dishes from the dishwasher. It was a slow task, and I stayed in bed without saying a word. About thirty minutes later, he tapped me on the shoulder and proudly stated, "Honey, I put all the dishes away for you." To see him so proud and content was a treasure! I had been patient enough not to stop him and simply returned the dirty dishes to the dishwasher in the morning. Afterward, I put a napkin under the top plates and bowls to find any unwashed ones faster.

Some nights just were not like the others. One particular night, I had settled into bed at 11 p.m. After twenty minutes, I heard the familiar creaking of the hall floor as Louis headed to the bathroom. I silently waited for him to return to bed so I could get up and turn off the water faucet. How thankful I was for that creaky floor! I shut off the water and dozed briefly until his next trot to the bathroom about twenty minutes later. This repeated ten or more times until he was sound asleep by around 3 a.m. Finally, I could get in three hours of sleep!

However, at 4 a.m., our fifty-pound dog pounced onto the bed, pushing me to get up. Abby was in panic mode, and Louis was sound asleep. Then I heard a sound that seemed only to go off during the night—that little sharp chirp from a smoke detector, telling me the battery was low. I had to determine which of the eight sensors it was and get the step ladder. Of course, the beep was much slower than I preferred, especially when trying to locate it. In the meantime, Abby wanted nothing to do with the process, and I hooked her up outside.

Finally, I removed the smoke detector and replaced the battery. Abby did not want to return, so I went out to persuade her that everything was fine. All done, or so I thought! As I headed back to bed, there was another chirp. Abby bolted for the outside door as I repeated the process with one less detector to check.

By this time, Louis was awake and up, wondering why so many lights were on. He helped me move the step ladder. As we returned to bed, I had to convince him it was not morning. After about thirty minutes, I was finally asleep when I heard Abby bark and realized I had left her outside. I tried apologizing to her as I dragged her into our attached garage. Then I discovered Louis had followed me to the door between our house and garage but had returned to bed and locked the door. I retrieved a spare key and returned to bed as Louis asked, "What took you so long?"

I often found myself at breaking point, longing to stop him and shout, "Just go to sleep!" The exhaustion and frustration were overwhelming. It took an immense reservoir of patience to stay silent in those moments. I masked my anger, even as I grappled with the stark reality of sleep deprivation. Finally, I resigned from my full-time job to care for Louis. I continued to take him to Daybridge, but the lack of sleep was taking a toll on my health.

Three weeks after resigning, I woke up with a strange tingle down my left arm that disappeared once I started moving around and took Louis to his day services place. Two days later, the same peculiar feeling in my left arm repeated. After taking Louis to DayBridge, I decided to get it checked out. I drove myself to a hospital emergency room and was admitted for an overnight stay with stress-induced cardiomyopathy, which is quite common among caregivers under severe stress and exhaustion. Stress cardiomyopathy is a condition leading to rapid and severe but reversible cardiac dysfunction and is caused by intense emotional or physical stress.

I did not know of any alternative care options to ease my burden, and now I felt at fault for having cardiomyopathy. I had planned to care for Louis at home and found it hard to accept that my strong body was failing. There were no suggestions from the hospital staff about what to do, although they seemed to approve that I had recently retired. The next day, I returned home—to where my husband's dementia could potentially harm me further.

My night stay in the hospital resulted in our son spending the night in our home with Louis. Paul asked how I got any sleep with his dad being up much of the night. Now our son understood my remarks about lack of sleep!

Three to four hours of very light sleep each day felt like a challenge I should be able to handle without complaint, but the difference in my physical strength just twenty-four hours after the stress-induced cardiomyopathy was staggering. Nevertheless, I had no thoughts of stopping and saying I couldn't manage such seemingly simple yet exhausting care.

Lou's dementia was rapidly worsening. I wanted to join conversations with family and friends with some freedom to ask for help, but Louis was always at my side. I often heard comments that he appeared to be doing well. While my husband was dozing in front of the TV, email was my way of sharing a few struggles with a compassionate friend. I hid the bruises on my body from when he grabbed at me or even swung an arm. No one would understand this was because of the dementia and that he had no clue what was happening or what he was doing.

Growing Responsibilities

As Louis' dementia deepened, my responsibilities grew. I became his protector, anchor to reality, and sole lifeline to a world slipping away from him. He relied on me for companionship and care but also more and more for his safety. Every day became a relentless marathon of vigilance. There were no private moments, no sanctuary to retreat to, and no respite from the constant demands of caregiving. When I was going to take a shower, I tried to get Louis to rest and pet Abby, but he would end up in the bathroom with me. He could take his own shower without help but kept asking, "Are you there?" His fear seemed to increase if I was not within sight.

I often relied on Abby to divert Louis when he was frustrated by being unable to complete simple household repairs like replacing a cartridge in a dripping faucet. She was great at cuddling and nudging him to pet her, and also with food spills: she stayed on high alert at mealtime! When Louis lay down for a nap on the sofa, Abby always managed to fit in with him.

However, I still longed to be alone for a few hours to run the snow blower without Louis walking behind me. Freedom to drive to the grocery store alone was only a dream. Neighbors did offer to get a few things, but I longed to shop without the shadowing of my husband. I yearned for those moments when someone would sit with Louis for an hour. Our friends seemed scared to offer help, and I was too ashamed to ask for it.

As is typical, I had taken over the management of our home. Sometimes, it meant taking over things my husband could no longer do, whether he was agreeable or not. Before the diagnosis of Alzheimer's, it had been an awkward burden when he acknowledged something he could not figure out and asked me to do it. However, with the diagnosis, he stopped trying and relied on my ability to do everything. I was not enthused!

One day, I got up on a twelve-foot ladder to snap screens over the roof gutters and asked Louis to hold the ladder, which he had done many times before. I was at the top of the ladder when he suddenly tried to move it over to the next section. That was a moment when I was glad about being heavy! When he shared with a good friend at church how hard it was to move the ladder with me at the top, the friend laughed and agreed it would be pretty tough. Without my asking, his friend completed the project a few days later while we were out. What a gift it was to come home and find it done!

The journey through dementia caregiving is a profound test of one's emotional and physical endurance. It required love and a reservoir of patience that ran deeper than I ever imagined. Each day and night presented its own unique set of challenges and heartaches. My experiences during those tumultuous times have left an indelible mark on my soul. As I navigated the sleepless nights and the bewildering behaviors, I clung to the hope that somewhere within the depths of my husband's fading memory, there was still a fragment of the person I loved, a fragment worth cherishing and protecting, no matter the cost.

The sensation of loneliness and emotional isolation that permeated my life when caring for Louis was one of the most heartbreaking parts of caregiving. I felt alone and disconnected even when he was physically present but unable to have meaningful conversations. As I yearned for the emotional connection we once had, I saw firsthand how carers' feelings of personal loss could result from their solitude.

This challenging journey blurred the lines between love, duty, and taking care of myself. I was unprepared for the exhaustion, helplessness, and anticipatory grief that accompanied caring for my increasingly dependent husband. The emotional toll was immense, and I needed outlets to process the complex feelings.

Often, I was too embarrassed to ask for advice about what was happening at home. I was in the turbulent emotional terrain caregivers face, not having enough information about what I needed in my unique situation or what might be available.

An Unwanted Role

I suddenly became my husband's caregiver, not by choice but because of the intimacy and commitment that are part of marriage. Being in this unwanted role of caregiver was hard. Caring for Louis differed significantly from the long-term care nursing career I had left two decades ago. Now, I was fearful I would make a mistake and not have the right things in order at the right time. Many carers worry that they will not properly care for their spouse or that they might pass away before their partner.

When the care recipient is our husband or wife, the people around us expect that we will take on the caregiving role. For those who are physically unable to do this or who become so during the caregiving journey, there remains a sense of responsibility often misunderstood by friends and family. In addition, the stress and physical toll on our bodies is part of a journey that no one else can fully comprehend. As a caregiver, it is hard to put our physical and emotional needs before those of our spouse. Another factor is that, despite still being legally married, we are no longer a part of the world of couples as we once were.

No two caregiving experiences are alike, even when dementia is the common thread. Each caregiver has a history, personality, and coping mechanisms. Similarly, the person with dementia is a unique individual with their own set of challenges, symptoms, and quirks. This intricate interplay of personalities and circumstances creates a dynamic that is impossible to fully grasp without walking precisely in the same shoes.

Challenges

For some, the heart-wrenching struggle lies in the difficult choice between continuing aggressive medical treatments or stopping these and transitioning their loved one to comfort care, also called palliative care. This comfort care may only qualify as hospice care if the person is not expected to live more than six months.

The rapid advances in medical technology and the desire of medical professionals to save and prolong life all add layers of complexity to this already agonizing decision-making process. We face a healthcare system prioritizing intervention and treatment.

There are profound ethical questions about the quality of life, personal autonomy, and the dignity of the person with dementia. Balancing the desire to provide the best possible care with the need to honor a person's wishes can be a dilemma for caregivers and family members alike.

In this situation, caregivers have untold emotional battles, like the instance of a farmer in a small Minnesota town with a population of five hundred. He cared for his wife with dementia and finally placed her in a nursing home. He was a well-known, kind man, but there was no plug to pull, so one day, as he visited, he shot his wife "To end her suffering." He knew his future would be in prison and waited for his arrest.

Caregivers and those who wish to help them must remember that each journey is unique and that for caregivers to express their feelings and concerns without incurring judgment is entirely acceptable. While others may offer well-intentioned advice or share their own experiences, it's crucial to recognize that no one can fully understand the intricacies of each situation.

Above all, a caregiver should honor their feelings and choices for the care of their spouse. Because there is no one-size-fits-all solution to dementia caregiving, the path they choose should reflect their individual needs and values and those of their loved one. By acknowledging the uniqueness of each caregiving journey, we can foster a more compassionate and understanding community that offers genuine support to those facing the challenges of dementia caregiving.

Imagine those challenges. To the overwhelmed caregiver, promises of support and guidance can sometimes feel like a mirage, failing to meet their unique needs and problems. They are inundated with trying to ensure their loved one's safety and well-being while caring for their home and other assets. Every day is filled with unexpected obstacles. They require new planks on the deck, but the information is often designed without awareness of their struggles and the particular dimensions of their bridge.

Caregivers need flexibility and relevant guidance from those who are empathetic, open-minded, and willing to listen without imposing their own beliefs or experiences. Caregivers need responses to their struggles that do not overload them with nonessential information. Meeting these needs might include details of caregiver support groups, guidance from healthcare professionals with expertise in dementia care, and how to consult with legal and financial experts who can provide tailored advice.

Such support can genuinely become the lifeline caregivers need as they navigate the challenges of dementia caregiving.

"Take Care of Yourself."—HOW?

As a caregiver, I became familiar with the admonition, "You need to take care of yourself." I would cringe and become very frustrated whenever someone shamed me with those words, rarely providing a tangible offer of help. It wasn't that I didn't understand the significance of looking after my well-being; it was because, all too often, people assumed that merely pointing out the need for self-care was enough to address my complex challenges. They gave me no idea of how they could help or what I could do. It is a scolding a caregiver does not need. At one evening event, I heard "You need to take care of yourself" more than eight times and left very angry. It was the last time we went there.

Many well-wishers failed to recognize the intricate layers of caregiving, which extended far beyond the simple notion of taking a break. The standard recommendations typically revolved around respite care, suggesting I should seek some temporary relief. However, those suggestions often lacked consideration for my practical realities.

One of the most important things was cost, which seemed unimportant to anyone but me. A friend gave me a number to call for 'free respite care'—an advertisement for a free respite care assessment—thinking that with an assessment, the care would also be free! My time was too valuable to make calls if no fees were listed in a brochure or website, so I immediately eliminated those that did not list prices or said to call for more information. Also, costs per day are often documented only for the lowest level of care needed.

Additional costs can include dealing with incontinence and providing incontinence products, dispensing meds, providing meals, and helping with eating and dressing. Many families are tasked with tending to various logistical aspects of the individual's life that may not be available at the facility and can incur additional costs. These might include managing clothing and personal belongings, ensuring access to or renting equipment such as wheelchairs and other mobility aids, and overseeing essential healthcare services, such as dental care and podiatry.

Moreover, there was an emotional aspect to consider. Would it be acceptable for me to be away from Louis? How would my absence impact his well-being, and would he feel comfortable with a strange caregiver? The potential for aggression or resistance from him added another layer of complexity that I couldn't ignore.

In response to these well-intentioned but vague suggestions to care for myself, I began to ask a simple question: "How?" I did this because when someone genuinely cared and was willing to offer assistance, they would come forward with something specific. I wanted to know if the offer was a genuine commitment to support me. I wanted to see if they considered the cost, the scheduling, and other details.

This experience taught me a valuable lesson I now share with others who want to help caregivers. Don't say, "Let me know if you need any help." Offer something concrete, such as, "Can I take your spouse (or both of you) out for pie and coffee this Wednesday afternoon?" Offer the caregiver multiple choices, such as inviting them over for supper, bringing them a casserole, or taking their loved one to an appointment for a haircut. Include the days you are available to do these things. Put your offer on paper or in an email, and request a response.

This approach demonstrates a genuine willingness to assist and eliminates the burden on the caregiver to remember the offer or to initiate the request for help. Organize a meal train using mealtrain.com. It could be set up for just once a week to give the caregiver a break.

The changes in the cognitive abilities of our spouses often happen in waves. There is no way to predict what will occur next or how we will respond. Consequently, caregivers should be prepared with two or three things they would like help with for those who offer to do so. I was not good at asking for help as I focused on the impossibility of getting more sleep. A neighbor knew how much I hated making meals and we were blessed with many evening meals at their house, which have continued despite Louis' absence.

Caregiving demands immense physical and emotional endurance. Caregiver fatigue can result from providing round-the-clock care, scheduling appointments, and dealing with dementia's unpredictable nature while also managing a home and sometimes full- or part-time employment. The continual changes and emotional whirlwinds are similar to the erosion from a river's current against the main supports of a bridge. I discovered that caring for a partner with dementia over the course of twenty years affected me more than I could ever have imagined. No matter whether you are a professional, a friend, or a family member of a caregiver of a spouse, the caregiver rarely shares the most challenging and often intimate moments of caregiving.

Less than a year after her husband died of Lewy Body dementia, I was sitting at a table with Daisy, a widow in her sixties, when she slumped over. She died a few hours later. Her caregiving had involved trying to get help and calling the police more than once. I could not imagine what she had been dealing with in their home. It was clear that caring for her husband had a tremendous impact on her health.

Her death influenced my desire to help current and future caregivers. That desire increased when I entered graduate school and began to read some of Dr. Joseph E. Gaugler's research at the University of Minnesota regarding mortality among caregivers. An article by Gaugler et al. (2018) that stood out was "Caregivers Dying Before Care Recipients with Dementia." I did not want to add my name to any statistics by dying a short time before or after the death of my husband.

Caregivers of spouses need help. We do not train ahead to be caregivers.

Protecting the Image of My Loved One

I was determined to fulfill my promise of "Till death do us part" by caring for my husband at home. Admitting that I could no longer do this was not an option I considered. Other caregivers had cared for their spouses with dementia at home until death. Despite the exhaustion and my deteriorating physical state, it took some significant changes in Louis before I decided to place him in a memory care facility.

Dementia caused inappropriate and embarrassing actions by him that I hid, knowing they contradicted information in the media. There were reports of assaults by caregivers in care facilities on residents with dementia, but the patient was never guilty. At times, I was shocked by his strength and unpredictable actions. What happened to me is an example of what a disease or a stroke can do to our brains and bodies. I continued to protect Louis' image of the quiet and caring person he had been, and I still have a sense of pride in what he lovingly accomplished.

I hid many things for a few years because I felt that, as Lou's wife, I would honor my promise to be with him until death. I yearned for the strength to care for him at home for the rest of his life—a strength I eventually no longer had.

What I hid, why I hid it, and how I tried to cope with what was available was not healthy or good. By shedding light on the hidden aspects of dementia caregiving, I hope to support others as they help strengthen the bridge, providing safe passage for caregivers like me to cross the turbulent waters of progressive dementia and other terminal conditions of care recipients.

Under Resources, you will find more information on steps for caregiver support.

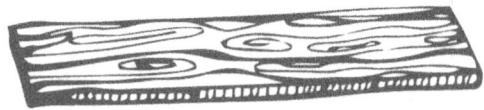

Hypersexuality and Aggression

I am sharing a few problematic things in hopes that you will become more aware of what caregivers do not tell and why I did not speak up. I hid signs of spousal abuse—scratches and bruises on my body—and was prepared to make excuses if anyone noticed. Some articles I had read put the caregiver at fault for failing to identify the triggers of aggressive behavior and not avoiding them. It was also very important to me for family and friends to see Louis as the kind person he always had been and not what the disease was doing to him. It was easy to hide because his behavior around them was perfect.

The progression of my loving husband's dementia brought with it a deepening fear that I could never have imagined. There were moments that I can only describe as terrifying when he would lunge at me, his grasp surprisingly strong as I struggled to release his clenched hands. It was as if his confusion and frustration had taken physical form. I would try to shield myself from being slapped at or grabbed while also preserving his dignity and safety. Dementia had inflicted these episodes upon him, turning him into someone I hardly recognized.

One of the most agonizing and least discussed aspects of being a caregiver was grappling with the issue of sexuality.

57

Caregivers rarely share about coping with the shameful sexual behaviors of their loved ones. It's an emotionally charged situation that left me feeling isolated and embarrassed. The situation became infinitely more complex as during the last months he was still at home, Louis began to grab me, trying to choke me and pin me to the floor, demanding I engage in sexual intercourse. This led to my being sexually abused by my own husband. When his sexual demands were not met, he became extremely frustrated and agitated. He had no comprehension of my attempts to refuse.

Other spouses have reported that hypersexuality is one of the most distressing symptoms to cope with. That is a mild way to put it, as it can also be dangerous. When a caregiver dies first, does anyone even think the wonderful spouse they were caring for may have strangled them? Yet, due to its sensitivity, this issue is often hidden and silenced. It is a tormenting aspect of caregiving that few are prepared to confront or discuss openly (Harel et al. 2022).

I struggled with a storm of emotions after these alarming developments. The shame and embarrassment were challenging, and I was unsure of how to react. I was afraid of being strangled; physically, I was much weaker than my husband, and it had been only five months since my heart failure. I did not want to give up on caring for Louis at home, but I knew my options for home care were not a good choice for my survival. However, because caregivers were said to be responsible for causing aggressive behaviors, and because there weren't any specific triggers, I always felt Lou's behavior was my fault and that I deserved the physical abuse. This was enhanced by the fact that I had always felt that to be an excellent wife, Louis would expect me to thrive on having a perfect home and entertaining with five-course meals on fancy dinnerware—like his mother. I had never thought of myself as good at cooking or entertaining because I grew up on a farm with no brothers, and outdoor work was my area of expertise.

The confusion I experienced was overwhelming; the embarrassment felt like evidence of my weakness. I carried on facing these complex and deeply distressing challenges, but my feelings of safety disappeared. I yearned for time to understand what was happening and to seek help or information about this frightening and unexpected dimension of Louis' symptoms, but the demands of caregiving left little room for research. It was a journey into the unknown, hoping my bridge would not completely collapse before I made it across.

I wished other caregivers had shared how they handled what they hid, just like the unseen cracks under the bridge. Would anyone believe me or even care about the heartbreaking effects of dementia? Everything I came across continued to focus on the caregiver as both stronger and the abuser, further intensifying my isolation and distress. I longed for help, but how would anyone know if I couldn't tell them what was happening?

There was no one to offer insights on what to do as I finally searched for nearby memory care facilities with openings. Most required down payments to save a bed, and I hadn't realized they had waiting lists.

Being harmed by my husband and subject to his aggressive sexual demands created a dissonance between the intimate partner he once was and the partner he had become. His cognitive decline meant he had trouble understanding the situation and responded with anxiety, unaware of the implications and impact of his behavior. As for me, living in and sharing such fluctuating dynamics, his abusive sexual behavior and my endeavors to preserve privacy in our relationship reduced me to an awkward and troublesome reality. Louis was now so different from the man I had married, the husband who had never hurt me or even raised his voice.

Healthcare professionals need to be aware of this silent phenomenon of spousal sexual assault, with a specific focus on the victimized caregiver and providing information on dementia-related hypersexuality and the accompanying caregiver's feelings of shame, embarrassment, confusion, and distress. This would, in turn, encourage open communication.

As a caregiver, I needed someone I could trust to confide in who was not family or a friend. I needed guidance on how I might move forward in safety for myself as I continued caring for my husband at home while looking at care facilities. Even before I was discharged from the hospital with cardiomyopathy, for my safety, I wished I had been told about the urgency of placing Louis in a care facility or had been warned about my own health. I had been too concerned about what others would think because he could still walk, was not incontinent, and seemed pleasant with friends and family.

Your loved one's specific care needs, preferences, and financial considerations change as the disease progresses. If you are depending on a home care agency, you must have plans in place should another pandemic occur or they close or no longer have personnel who are able or licensed to care for your spouse. Remember that if you hire someone yourself, you become an employer and will have payroll taxes to pay and file.

I think of how caregivers live inside homes that can become like prisons, trying the best they can to care for a loved one. Not even family members know how silence can hurt. If you are a caregiver, know it is very easy to focus on your loved one's needs and not your own. Getting help or accepting any offer of help is as complex as making the call and admitting we can no longer survive caring for our spouse at home.

At this point, I had little desire to end my life but also little reason to feel my life was worth living.

Help at Home Can Result in More Work for the Caregiver

Friends and family may be quick to think that having help with caregiving at home provides caregivers some rest. It is often the opposite. Many times, having help ends up being more work for the caregiver and incurs significant expenses compared to the cost of placing a loved one in memory care.

Even with twenty-four-hour care, the caregiving spouse has the additional responsibility of having a backup plan when there are no-shows or if there should be other pandemics, such as COVID-19. There is a progressive increase in laundry that can pile up like rocks in a riverbed. There may be future needs for special equipment like a hospital bed, wheelchair, shower chair, stair lift, and a soaking tub for dirty laundry; renovations of the home may be needed by widening doorways. There could be more groceries needed because making meals that may need to be puréed for your loved one might be different from the food you or any hired help want to eat.

I desperately needed sleep, but no agency could provide a caregiver willing to stay through those darkest hours, turn off a water faucet every twenty minutes, and leave at 3 a.m. when Louis was finally asleep for the rest of the night.

I also simply could not fathom the thought of a stranger stepping into our home and taking over Louis' care. It felt like stepping on a partially broken plank on that bridge. Perhaps one of the most daunting concerns was the potential for Louis to react negatively to the presence of someone he didn't know. The fear of aggression or resistance loomed, making hiring in-home help even more unsettling. I did not want to invite strangers into this turbulence.

In addition, this was also before COVID-19, when there was already a massive shortage of home healthcare workers.

There are so many other things to consider when your loved one is at home: medical appointments, medication management, haircuts, podiatry, dental hygiene, and a need for easy-to-change clothing like sweatpants and other clothes with no buttons or zippers. In rural areas, deliveries are often left at mailboxes. A caregiver may need to walk a quarter mile to obtain a frozen gallon of milk while leaving their spouse alone. Having a ramp into your home for a wheelchair and a vehicle that you can transfer your loved one into is essential because there are times you may be alone. Making appointments takes extra time to make sure that wherever you are going, the place can accommodate your spouse. With all the automated systems for scheduling, few offer the opportunity to talk to a live person and make appropriate arrangements.

The decision to transition from home caregiving to a care facility was fraught with heartache and uncertainty. I grappled with feelings of inadequacy and shame, torn between my desire to provide the best care for Louis and the overwhelming toll that caregiving had taken on my well-being. It was a pivotal crossroads in our journey, requiring immense courage and strength.

As I reflect on the profound caregiving journey, one sentiment resonates deeply: the yearning for privacy from others. Over the years, I've encountered individuals who, much like me, naturally gravitate toward leading private lives. Our homes serve as our refuge, offering solace and comfort amid our challenges. We hold our family's stories close to our hearts. In a world where support may come in the form of hired caregivers, compassionate church members, kind neighbors, or even well-meaning siblings, the idea of opening our doors and sharing the intricacies of our lives—whether they pertain to our aging loved ones or to us—can be disconcerting. The intimacy of our spaces and the vulnerability of our circumstances converge to create a longing for privacy.

The sanctuary of our homes, where our daily lives unfold, carries immense emotional weight. It is where memories are etched into the walls, laughter and tears have left their indelible marks, and love and care have been guiding forces. It's only natural that we instinctively want to preserve the sanctity of these spaces. I was not willing to break many boundaries I had in our home.

Finding the balance between privacy and assistance is a complex endeavor that requires thoughtful consideration of our needs as caregivers and the needs of our loved ones. It involves setting boundaries that protect our privacy and opening the door to compassion and care that can lighten our burden by allowing others to share and help us. In moments of vulnerability and openness, we may find the solace and strength to carry on.

Though it is admirable to want to care for a loved one at home, there came a time when I needed to be aware of my limits for the benefit of both myself and Louis. I did not want to make that decision and hoped someone would suggest it was time to place him in memory care. But no one asked if the caregiving was getting to be too much for me. It was my decision alone to make.

It is easy today to look back and realize that, at the time, I did not know how or what I needed—beyond sleep! Now, I can suggest how to help other caregivers.

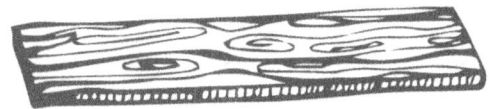

Do You Think My Loved One Is Ready to Go to Memory Care?

As it was for me, moving their spouses out of their homes is a decision caregivers may hope someone else, such as a doctor, family member, or day services staff, will make for them.

One day, I was given notice by DayBridge that they would only be able to care for Louis for another week as he was becoming aggressive with their staff. The manager also shared her serious concerns about my safety and why I needed to act immediately, which I did.

I needed to hear that concern and not have to ask a professional, "Do you think Louis is ready to go to memory care?" Other caregivers have shared how they would ask doctors, nurses, social workers, and others they looked up to, and the familiar response was, "I don't know." That response is so disheartening to a caregiver! You may be the only person they can look to for advice.

Have you ever asked why they asked you? If a caregiver asks if it is time for their loved one to be placed in memory care, ask the caregiver if the care is getting to be too much for them. You are not giving them your thoughts but guiding them to focus on their health and maybe think about their response. It is easy to say, "I don't know," but that can feel as if you don't care. It is a choice the caregiver needs to make, but can you say five more simple words? "I don't know—but why do you ask?" This could be your only chance to have them focus on themselves and not their loved ones. You may hear that they are on overload, both physically and emotionally. Reflect back on what they just said and encourage them to think about it. This is your opportunity to save a caregiver's life!

I felt my heart could not handle more stress at home. But I also felt that if I shared this, I would be admitting how weak I was and someone might ask more about what exactly was happening there. However, I ruled out providing care around the clock within the confines of our home; there was no way to predict how long it would be required, and our split-level house was not suited for a wheelchair. Each twist and turn would bring new challenges to compound the overwhelming stress already threatening to drown me.

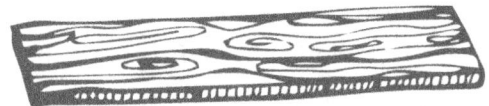

Focus on the Caregiver's Well-Being

No one knows the exact moment at which a bridge will collapse. The extreme stress that accompanies dementia caregiving is like the eroding supports of that rotting wood bridge over the Dementia River. Dementia erodes the caregiver's resilience and can hide their struggles beneath the surface from the view of others. The weight of these challenges leads some caregivers to unhealthy coping mechanisms, like alcohol and drugs, which further weaken their bridge. Caregivers rarely have the time or willingness to share their hidden battles. As we've discussed, protecting the privacy of a marriage is a big contributing factor to this.

It is vital that others help make the bridge safe, enabling caregivers and those they care for to traverse the tumultuous waters of dementia with strength and resilience. In order to do this, it is critical to raise awareness from the caregiver's point of view rather than that of those who may think they know what the caregiver needs. It is only by discovering what is often hidden by the caregiver that we can reinforce the supports, replace rotting wood, and provide a solid bridge to those on this challenging path.

The decision to place a spouse in a full-time care facility should focus on the caregiver rather than the care recipient. I needed to stay alive and mentally capable of being a care advocate for my husband. I was familiar with his care and protection. I was the one who would be handling the financial provisions and care decisions. I was the one who knew he wanted quality of life and not to have it artificially extended when he might be suffering or no longer knew or responded to people.

Focus on the Caregiver

- **Physical Limitations:** Caregiving can be physically demanding, especially when a spouse's health needs escalate. Lifting, assisting with mobility, and attending to various daily tasks can all affect a caregiver's physical health. Ignoring their physical limitations can lead to injuries, chronic health issues, and an inability to provide adequate care. Caregivers must understand there's no shame in seeking professional assistance when the physical demands become too much to handle.
- **Emotional Limitations:** Caregiving is emotionally taxing as well. It can bring about feelings of stress, anxiety, shame, and burnout. Caregivers may feel torn between their spouse and caregiver roles, leading to internal conflict. Recognizing these emotional limitations is essential for maintaining the caregiver's mental health.
- **Quality of Care:** Striving to provide care beyond one's physical and emotional capacity can compromise the quality of care given to the spouse. When a caregiver is overstressed or exhausted, their ability to make sound decisions and provide compassionate care diminishes. This

affects not only the caregiver but also the well-being of the spouse.

- **Seeking Help Is a Sign of Strength:** Caregivers need to understand that seeking professional care and considering alternative care settings, like a nursing home or a memory care facility, is not a sign of failure. It's a sign of strength and taking responsibility. It shows that the caregiver is prioritizing their spouse's well-being and safety above all else.
- **Open Communication:** Caregivers of spouses cannot rely on their loved one with dementia to tell them what to do. A supportive family is good, but ultimately, care needs to focus on the caregiver's well-being. Moving a spouse out of the home is usually the most difficult decision a caregiver will ever make.

Family members may fail to agree, or they may help encourage placement, but when it is time to stop caring for a spouse at home, the focus needs to be on the caregiver. Because the caregiver is often exhausted and focused only on their loved one, they may also need help admitting they can no longer manage home care. Respect and support them! Remind them it is okay to forget any promises, such as "I will never put you in a nursing home," and realize the importance of staying alive and adjusting to being a care advocate for their loved one in a care facility.

In Minnesota, memory care is licensed differently from assisted living. Staffing ratios are higher. Memory care staff have certifications in memory care with frequent updates and refresher courses, and depending on the level of care, most have training that exceeds that of nursing home staff.

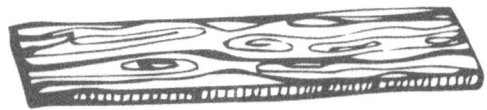

Care Facilities and Memory Care Choices

Care Facilities

Many folks do not have the opportunity to check out different facilities. Unexpected hospital admission for a broken bone or sudden surgery often involves the patient being placed in a rehabilitation facility that has an opening and can handle the necessary care. While advocating for your hospitalized loved one, there may be only a few days to find a place that has an opening and to find out whether they take Medicare if your spouse was receiving Social Security benefits.

As we discussed earlier, Medicare is limited to twenty days of complete coverage, then eighty days during which the patient is responsible for the copay. Beyond one hundred days in a licensed care facility is not covered by Medicare or health insurance.

This is also a good time for the caregiver to acknowledge they cannot care for the patient at home anymore and refuse to take them home. The facility where they are currently is required to find them a place. The caregiver must stand firm and not take their loved one home even for a few more days. Taking them home removes the pressure from the discharging facility, and the caregiver will have to make all the arrangements, which can take months and even a year or more.

Trying to compare the costs of different places is almost impossible. Some places list only room and board, with care and dispensing of medication considered extras. Others list a level of care package without including the cost of room and board.

Transitioning to a higher level of care within a facility may mean relocating the individual to a different room or area with more staffing to handle their evolving care needs. This adjustment can be emotionally challenging for both the caregiver and the resident, as it often signifies a significant shift in their relationship and daily routines, plus an increase in cost.

There are other options to consider when dealing with medical issues and extra charges for care. Different levels of memory care have different staffing ratios. Some facilities are not prepared to handle hospice care, so they send residents to a hospital. Not all hospice teams are trained to manage the final stage of dementia care. They are used to working with people who may be able to communicate relatively clearly almost until the end.

Memory Care

If dementia is advanced, most memory care facilities are equipped and qualified to deliver medical care together with dementia care. In Minnesota, staffing-to-patient ratios are highest for memory care. As the disease progresses, more care is needed, and costs rise.

When comparing costs for memory care facilities, it's essential to consider various factors to be sure you're making an informed decision. It is helpful to have some recommendations from families of loved ones with dementia.

Your spouse's dementia may not follow every stage you have read about, whether you are trying to determine the stage of the disease using three, five, eight, or ten stages as their disease progresses. You may think, for example, that since they remember people's names, they are only in the early stages, but some may know who you are even in the final stage. Some facilities send residents who can no longer swallow to a hospital where extension of life is the usual focus, keeping them alive with what may be painful procedures rather than focusing on comfort care.

Memory care is specifically designed for those suffering from many types of diseases that cause dementia, such as Alzheimer's, Lewy body dementia, vascular dementia, frontotemporal dementia, and over 120 others.

To me, it seemed selfish to cling to Louis and not be able to let him go to his heavenly home. I wanted to find somewhere that would provide palliative care, where the focus is on pain management and not prolonging any suffering with the disease.

I also looked for facilities where there was no such thing as a 'bed-ridden patient'. I wanted provision for residents to be out in the common areas and not alone in their rooms, as well as to be able to eat in common dining areas.

Another focus of mine was how a place adapted to the progression of a resident's dementia and that it did not use cost-cutting measures like lumping all stages together for activities. If I were being admitted and had any sense of my surroundings, I would not want to be seated with those in the final stage of dementia; I'd want to be with others who were like me and with whom I could communicate or do things, like playing games. Being close to home, staffing ratios, and costs were also important to me.

Moving to memory care is a crucial step in ensuring that the care provided to a loved one is of the highest quality and that the caregiver's well-being is safeguarded. I must stress again that deciding to transition your loved one to memory care when necessary is an act of love and responsibility, showing a commitment to the best possible outcome for both you and your spouse. I had underestimated the importance of respecting my limitations, both physically and emotionally.

It is very difficult to live with the feeling that we should have cared for our loved ones at home for even a few more weeks or months longer. They often seem too well when we move them out of their home. Yes, the care will differ, but we must acknowledge that the disease's progress will require higher staffing ratios and greater care than we can possibly provide.

Under Resources, you will find more information on memory care.

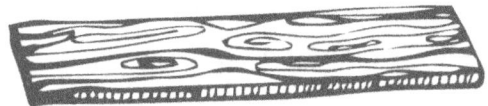

Placement in Memory Care

Fourteen years after his initial symptoms of dementia began as 'depression' and two years after he was diagnosed with final-stage Alzheimer's disease, I felt I could not handle Louis beyond a few more days and called our son, who provided great support as we immediately attempted to place Louis in a full-time care facility.

My most agonizing decision was making the call, admitting I needed to place my husband in memory care. The shame and grief, sadness, and gnawing feeling of failure weighed heavily on me, but I finally recognized it was a necessary step for the safety and well-being of both of us.

I called the nearby facility where I had left a downpayment for a room. Before admitting Louis, they required a registered nurse on their staff to do an assessment. She went to the day services facility Louis had attended on weekdays to determine what he was like around other people, including the staff. In her brief time there, she discovered he had shown signs of sudden agitation that was rapidly escalating, and he had recently slapped one of the employees.

In addition, Louis would first need a ten-day gerontological-psychological evaluation as a hospital patient, which was covered by Medicare. This took two months of waiting, and during that time, his behavior made an unexpected change as he became more sexually aggressive. He always seemed so sleepy that I hadn't thought he would have bursts of energy in any form.

My patience and strength were gone. My bridge was shaking and crumbling. Planks were tumbling to the river below. I was about to collapse and let the river current take me under, but he was my hubby, and I still wanted to hang on to him.

When I drove Louis to the hospital, I did not tell him what was happening; I just said a different doctor needed to see him, so he had no idea it was a hospital. It was a heartbreaking drive, knowing he would never live at home again.

During those ten hospital days, he was snowed under with more medication. Then, before he could be discharged from the hospital to memory care, I was told by the memory care facility that they could not take him because of his behavior problems. However, the nurse from that facility, who had done his assessment, immediately stepped in to help me without any charge.

She could find only one place within a thirty-mile radius of our home that had an opening in their behavioral care unit and would take him. Wealshire of Bloomington, MN, a large memory care facility with a behavioral unit and four other units based on different levels of care, seemed rather high class, but I had no other choice. It was also twenty miles away.

I was able to make all the arrangements that same day and drove there to put a few clothes in Louis' room. Then I fetched him from the hospital. He was happy to be 'going home' and never asked about the forty-five-mile route I took, telling him we needed to make a stop on the way.

The overwhelming stress and load of shame were terrible! During the drive, I fought back the tears as Louis became interested in the seatbelt and tried to open the car door at 60 mph. I finally got him to settle down and thought about how I had turned down another caregiver in my support group who offered to come with me. Now I could see it had not been a good idea to do that drive without help.

I walked Louis into Wealshire, where he would be for the last six years of his life. We made it to his room, where the staff warmly welcomed him and distracted him with a dish of ice cream. This allowed me to easily slip out, take care of some more paperwork, and be told the plans for the next three days. I was to rest and not visit during that time.

That evening, my neighbors invited me over for supper while I shared the most challenging day of our married life. No matter how exhausted I was, I needed a healthy meal and caring listeners.

Each morning, the Wealshire staff sent an email update, including any questions they had. One included a form for his life story and a request that I attach a few photos. All this information would familiarize the staff with his past and our family.

Before I left after my first visit, a life enrichment staff member was sitting at a table with Louis and two other men. He asked them what kind of jobs or professions they would like to learn more about and focus on those, not what they had done prior for a living. The first man said he wanted to drive a submarine that would stay above water. The next wanted to be a groundskeeper to drive the carts on a golf course. Louis said, "Electrician," and then added, "Because Dwight and Bill and Horst taught me at church." The staff member looked at me for clarification. It was special to tell him Louis was right and that the guys he'd mentioned were not pastors. Louis had learned from them during our church work days and, for many years, had done well with what they taught him. I left as he was asked what he had wired, and he said, "The barn at the farm and offices and compressors." His mind was clear for that moment of good memories.

During that visit, he never mentioned going home, but the next time, he asked, "What did I ever do to you to deserve this?" It was his last ever clearly expressed statement! I could only try, while fighting back the tears, to say, "You have a disease and need help I cannot give you right now." On a snowy day six years before his death, Louis' last understandable words to me were, "Hi Abby." At least he identified me as family, though I was sure I did not look quite like our dog!

The dementia-only care facility he was in was indeed excellent. I did not need to take him out of the facility for anything. No appointments, haircuts, podiatry—nothing! Everything was in-house. I never once worried about the care he was receiving, as it surpassed my wildest expectations and proved infinitely superior to what I could ever have offered him within the confines of our home.

Sometimes, on my phone in the morning, there were mandatory notifications about significant events, such as Louis taking a roll out of bed during the night with no apparent injury. (He rolled onto a special floor mat two inches lower than his bed, as side rails or restraints are illegal.) Being consulted about any changes in medications felt respectful to me. The goal was to reduce his dosages of medication to a point where he was not so drowsy all the time.

Recognizing and respecting my physical and emotional limitations as a caregiver had been critical to providing the best care for Louis. As I recount these moments, I am reminded of the delicate balance between the desire to provide unwavering care and the acknowledgment of one's limitations.

While I knew deep down that relinquishing my role at home as the primary caregiver had been necessary, I found it agonizingly difficult to let go. It wasn't merely about acknowledging my limitations; it was the emotional entanglement that kept me tethered to the role.

The first two months Louis was away from home were some of my most challenging days. I had not anticipated what it would be like to have no job. Was I needed by anyone anymore? Comparisons gnawed at me, each ripple of doubt questioning my ability to cope. How did other caretakers manage the bridge gracefully from the sanctuary of their homes while, even with my background in long-term care, I struggled?

I must make it clear that I was grateful no longer to be solely responsible for the burden of Louis' care. Despite his physical health, his dementia progressed very fast during those first two months at the Wealshire of Bloomington. During the second month, balance issues made it impossible for him to walk, and he was no longer able to manage eating utensils, though he could eat finger food. He was already almost totally deaf. This had been established a year earlier, and I was told at the time that hearing aids wouldn't help with the type of hearing loss he had.

Louis' speech disappeared, his pupils were dilated, and his eyes appeared empty. By the third month, he was unable to feed himself finger food, though he continued eating when a spoon touched his teeth while he was being fed. Of course, these rapid changes required more staff care.

There was a secured outdoor patio on Louis' unit, and that first December was warm with only a touch of snow. A special request from the staff was, "Please bring Abby." Abby loved to visit and took in all the petting from Louis and several other residents. She only objected to entering the elevator, where a voice from the ceiling said, "Floor one, floor two." After her first elevator ride, she made her preference for using stairways very well-known. When residents noticed a dog near them, there were happy faces. Pets were like heroes to most of them, and our pet liked to be shared with every person in sight. I brought Abby many more times, but within those first two months, Louis stopped responding to her, even when she pushed and nudged him.

Later, I noticed that some residents in the final stage unit seemed comforted by robotic cats that purred and turned their heads when petted. One resident who could still talk had a moment of clarity and told me her cat was not real, but she still liked to pet him all day because she had cats in her home. It was so nice to hear her reminisce and be happy!

Three months after his placement in memory care, Louis was moved out of the behavioral care unit to the final stage dementia unit of the facility, where he would remain until his death six years later. The move was all taken care of by the staff without any need for me to be there.

My husband, while unresponsive, was up every day in his wheelchair. This daily mobility likely contributed to the absence of pressure sores, underlining the importance of residents not being confined to their beds. Movement and circulation significantly maintained overall comfort, particularly in the residents' limbs.

I dreaded a future of watching Louis simply be alive. Despite his vegetative state, I had no choice but to let his body live on. In a different lifetime, we had discussed how we both wanted quality of life and not length or quantity. We desired comfort care only and had opted for do-not-resuscitate (DNR) and do-not-intubate (DNI) orders, as well as no antibiotics or anything that might prolong life, like protein drinks, once our minds were gone or pain was beyond the control of medication. But I had no control on Louis' behalf, as in our world of modern medicine, the focus is on prolonging life rather than focusing on its quality.

Once the separation took place, those around me seemed to think I could now get some rest and sleep. However, caregiving had not ended when Louis entered the memory care facility; it simply changed. Now I noticed a lot more to take care of than just my husband.

I had put off self-care and neglected my health as Louis's care became my top priority. For ten years, it had not been important to go for a physical or have my teeth cleaned. I had home upkeep to do. Church and social groups had changed because I had missed many gatherings and conversations. If I were to return, it would be without my mate.

I had lost a large portion of my identity. Where did I fit now? With couples or with singles? Also, my interests had changed. I did not want to be entertained or be on the go all the time. I had to navigate the changed interests, the loss of friends, and the paradox of still being married but no longer a couple. A group of widowed women from our church managed to include me in their activities and understood my isolation and need for socialization, but though I am thankful for their persistence, I struggled to feel I belonged with them.

I resented the question, "How is Louis?" and having to respond week after week and year after year with, "No change." All the time Louis was in memory care, it seemed that no one asked how I was doing or how I was handling the stress! No one was entertaining the possibility of helping me. Again, I was told, "Take care of yourself," while I did my best under circumstances others could not understand. They were not in my shoes, in our home, or standing alongside my unresponsive husband! One exception was my backyard neighbors who, while Louis was still at home, would often invite us over for supper and have continued ever since to have me over on short notice. They are incredible listeners without pushing suggestions, demonstrating unique ways of helping me know I am not forgotten.

As this lonely memory care journey continued, the stress continued to take a toll on my health. Being part of Louis' care team and being consulted about actions to be taken did help give me some sense of purpose, but my life had changed profoundly. Even if the relief from direct caregiving and not feeling safe at home had ended, I now understood those words of support group members: "It only gets worse."

COVID-19

Amid the challenging backdrop of the COVID-19 pandemic, the high-quality care provided to Louis continued to shine as a beacon of hope and support. During the shutdown, I received general daily updates via email, a lifeline that proved invaluable in keeping me informed about his condition. This practice of regular communication from the director of nursing also meant concerned primary caregivers didn't interrupt staff with phone calls, and we were assured we would be contacted if there were any changes in their health or care.

As I reflect on those months, I must admit that I felt relief in not being able to visit Louis. It lifted the weight of the comparisons I often made with other spouses.

One particularly poignant moment during the pandemic stands out in my memory. A nurse, believing that Louis was in his final hour, summoned me to his bedside at 2 a.m. With the required protective garb, I remained by his side for two days.

Wearing protective clothing and a mask and shield gave me a profound appreciation for the staff who wore such gear daily, most working sixteen-hour shifts with more than their standard workload of residents. I admired their dedication and resilience. The decision to have me come to what appeared to be the end of my husband's life demonstrated the tremendous concern and respect the staff had for the immediate family.

Despite his ashen face and motionless form when I arrived, Louis stabilized. I had mixed feelings as we put him in his wheelchair to change his bed. He drank a glass of water and was fed two bowls of applesauce. I hid some disappointment, knowing that this extension of his life without any measures beyond keeping him comfortable meant the possibility of more suffering for Louis and more struggle trying to maintain my health.

Unfortunately, many families did not share the same fortune during the COVID-19 pandemic. The help at home that some caregivers needed was no longer available. Those using home services provided by a county or other staffing agency found their help was gone. People in rural areas seemed willing to help each other but were slower in adapting to technology and protective devices, including masks.

Abiding by state mandates with frequent daily changes and providing care amid staff shortages was nothing short of an extraordinary commitment of nursing staff and those who provided the essential resources to keep the facility running. It was a challenging time, but it also showcased the remarkable strength of the human spirit and the boundless capacity for care and compassion in the face of adversity.

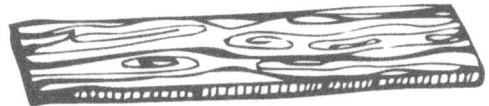

Guilt and Shame

I continued to fail at caregiving. Partly, this was because I found it very hard to visit Louis frequently and compared myself to other spouses who stayed many hours every day. I, on the other hand, did not have a regular schedule for visiting, though I would often go to feed him during meal times, and I found that the twenty-mile drive helped me settle down before and after visits. The family could visit anytime, and the primary contact/caregiver always had the most recent door codes, one for the front entrance and another for entering the unit. It felt like I had no excuse.

That several caregivers in our support group still cared for spouses and other loved ones at home continued to remind me that here I was, an RN who had failed. As a result, I felt I did not deserve any positive comments about how I had cared for Louis at home. My feelings of hopelessness and failure were hard to bear, and I was physically weak from the cardiomyopathy and years of very little sleep.

I had assumed that once Louis was in memory care, there would be much less stress and more sleep, but that assumption was more like a distant dream. I could not get a good night's rest, and even Abby was restless the first hours of bedtime.

I still listened for the creaky floor and running water faucet and realized that I was navigating a now-ingrained habit of constant alertness and readiness to address any potential concerns or emergencies that might arise. Over a year after Louis had left our home, I still heard every little sound during the night. I would listen to the refrigerator going on and off, the furnace starting six times, and Abby pacing up and down the stairs.

I realized that even when Louis was no longer at home, caregiving was still changing me. Some of those changes made me a better person, and I try to look at this caregiving experience and see the good in what happened. But as soon as I started thinking I should have kept Louis at home for longer or that caring for him at home had not been that tough, the guilt tended to return. My emotions were often numb and still often are. Then the thoughts would come crashing back, and I felt how ugly, selfish, degrading, resentful, and angry I was. Most of the time, I didn't know what triggered it, but I was too exhausted and frustrated to feel I could do much about it. My anger at the little things I had overlooked stuck for hours and days instead of minutes.

Many times during the six years Louis was in memory care, I wondered what was so great about looking after my own health. I was now only a care advocate; my job as a caregiver at home was done. I was at a new point in life. I did not know the future. To handle the guilt of having a hubby in the last stage of Alzheimer's is beyond what others will understand.

Guilt led to more depression: the guilt of not being able to care for him at home, the guilt of my body failing from the stress-induced illness, the guilt of having fun, the guilt of enjoying time alone, the guilt of working on projects alone, the guilt of making decisions alone, the guilt of reacting negatively to what seemed to be just about everything, the guilt over my lack of concentration to the point of avoiding things like book clubs or Bible studies, the guilt of going to the farm alone, and the guilt of having so many up and down moods. Financial considerations became increasingly complex as well. It felt as if my brain was being stretched in every way possible, but it was good for me to be focusing away from hands-on care.

In her book, *Loving Someone With Dementia*, Dr. Pauline Boss uses the term 'ambiguous loss' to describe grief that has no end (Boss 2011). As a caregiver, I felt the ambiguous loss of my husband, who for over six years was physically present but mentally absent. This was a never-ending grieving for him, and it forced me to confront a new and confusing relationship in which he didn't know who I was and had no ability to speak, hear, or even see properly.Among Older Widows and Widowers.

Unsuitable Coping Skills - Beer Bingeing and Suicidal Thoughts

I missed the love that had felt so strong when Louis and I worked together. Even when he could no longer help me, I still sensed his feelings of helplessness and desire to do so. Louis' dementia was a significant loss not only to him but also to me. During the evenings, it was easy to mask my depression by bingeing on beer when I was sure I would not need to drive anywhere the rest of the night.

Louis' qualifying and not qualifying for hospice was the most difficult for me, and it happened five times in six years. There were moments when I felt I could not go on, and the best thing would be to end my life. Who cared? Was I even needed or wanted anymore?

I find it hard to explain the feelings of watching Louis live on. I felt helpless, especially not knowing if he was feeling pain that he could not convey to anyone. Even though I never harbored any apprehension about his care, not knowing if he was suffering was heartbreaking, and I continued to struggle.

It did not feel right to be hoping for his death, but my deep concern about his possible suffering was not something I could explain to others. Five years later, in his final days, when he could no longer swallow and therefore couldn't eat, oral drops of morphine were routinely given. It made no sense to have it ordered to be dispensed as needed since he couldn't say when he needed it. This was a blessing in my hope that he wasn't suffering.

I could never totally 'let go' of Louis because of our marriage vows. I felt love for him that I could not fully rationalize. He was still my husband, and I chose to honor my commitment. How I wanted back that person who was once so lovable!

I missed having someone to bounce things off, like setting the water softener that needed recycling, mulching the leaves, or pointing out the chatter in the piston of our lawnmower, which meant only one thing—it was about to croak. When a spouse dies, it is final, and those little remarks are gone—but Louis was not dead, so I had the guilty feeling of not relying on him and instead needing to get help from others or do it myself. A mind with dementia might have died, but his body remained alive.

Beer was a handy item, and on many evenings, I ended up drinking several cans. This worsened every time Louis stabilized and was taken off hospice care. I was too exhausted and overwhelmed to seek assistance, yet I realized the dangers of substance abuse and self-harm.

Many friends assumed I should feel good not to have Louis at home anymore. Others assumed I would have extra time to go to different events with them as though there were no more worries—as if I no longer had an excuse! I would be asked to join them, starting with the phrase, "Now that you don't have Louis at home, you will be able to come ...." Because my schedule seemed open, it did not mean I was ready to handle an event I had previously attended with Louis.

It also seemed as if nobody understood that I needed time to catch up on all the health-related things I had put off for around ten years. I was worried about not regaining my strength after the cardiomyopathy. In fact, my heart may never be back to what it should be. As I tried to catch up on those years of ignoring my health concerns, there would be the usual scolding from the professionals involved about not being seen for so long and dropping medication renewals that required appointments. My primary physician was gone, as was my dentist. When a new dental clinic called saying they were missing four years of records from my previous dentist, they seemed surprised when I replied that there were none. And it wasn't just me; our home was also in need of some care.

Now that I was beginning to see what had been neglected at home, I was so exhausted that I didn't care if anyone saw my messy house. What once seemed important had changed to "Forget it." I had filtered out only the crucial things and had little or no energy to get my house back in order. Others around me may have thought they had experienced stress, but they had no idea what this stress felt like. They also didn't understand that I didn't know how much more stress I could take.

Two years after he became a memory care resident, I wrote: "Louis does not appear to know anyone, and his eyes appear blank with no constricting of his pupils. He may have some arthritic pain, does not seem to have sight or hearing, does not talk, but can still chew whole food fed to him. He opens his mouth when a spoon of food touches his teeth. His days are spent out in the common areas in his wheelchair. My most significant concern is that Louis be free of pain and suffering. The care is fantastic!"

Regardless of the quality of care, it was difficult for me to watch Louis when I didn't know if he was comfortable. After my visits, I would come home exhausted to that misguided relaxation of drinking beer late into the night.

My support group for caregivers met twice a month. It was a meeting I was not about to miss. Being with others as they cross their bridges and listening with encouragement is rewarding. The facilitator was a fantastic listener and had an amazing way of allowing us to help each other and see a purpose in what we were learning from our own experiences. She is a social worker who continues to work in adult day services.

However, and it bears repeating, no one else knows what your journey is like because every caregiver is different, and so is every spouse with dementia. No matter who tried to alleviate my feelings of shame, I had regrets. Could I have lasted another month caring for him at home? Were there some bad decisions I would make differently if I had another chance? The toughest part was accepting that I would not get a second chance.

Another area that distressed me was figuring out how to plan our finances based on how long Louis might live. At first, three years in the memory care facility seemed plenty to plan for, but he was there six years! I had no idea how long I could hold on, not just emotionally and physically but also financially.

I studied the regulations for applying for Medicaid (Medical Assistance in MN) at length, thinking I would need to apply if he lived longer. Taking the cash value of our life insurance policies so there was nothing left did not seem fair, as the life insurance companies would benefit from what we had paid over many years. A neighbor lost a five hundred thousand dollar life insurance policy because he had to 'spend down' to qualify for Medicaid for his wife and use the policy's cash value for her care, which was about $55,000.00. I think of that as a $445,000 loss to him and a gain for the insurance company. He can keep their house and live there until his death, on which the state has a lien and against which it will claim back what was paid for the care of his wife.

To qualify for Medicaid, the five-year look-back at all our financial records resulted in many findings that seemed unfair to the healthy spouse. Those with low income and minimal assets receive free care for their loved ones, while we were losing all that we had earned and saved for our retirement. I continue to feel that others in a similar situation are penalized for being married.

Amid all this pressure, drinking was easy to hide, and I later learned when reading an article in the Journal of the American Geriatrics Society on binge drinking how common it is for older people to acquire addictions to alcohol and other substances (Han et al. 2019). Fortunately, I was able to admit the bingeing to a therapist and worked on better coping skills.

Little things often made a difference to the stress I was coping with. It did help to know I was not forgotten even though I was no longer engaging in activities and events. I needed to know that, no matter how hard it was to respond. An email or text, "Just thinking of you," was encouraging, something I did not have to reply to but which told me I was still remembered. It allowed me to share if I desired to. Writing an email was often a stress releaser.

Helpful things have been friends inviting me over for a very informal meal, going out to eat, or helping blow out my snow plow ridge if I didn't get it done. To this day, I usually blow out my neighbors' ridges during daytime snow so they can make it into their garages when coming home from work. I remember how special it was to come home to a cleared driveway. It was one thing Louis could still do while at home alone after he was laid off from his work.

My hubby was a great handyman, and now, as I learn to ask, my neighbors are giving me that gift of helping. Several times, a neighbor noticed I had just returned from visiting Louis and said, "Come over for supper." It was often the spontaneous things that helped me deal with stress, depression, loneliness, loss, expenses, and other struggles, even the drinking.

For more information on this topic, see the section later in this book: Addictions and Suicides Among Older Widows and Widowers.

Seeking Therapy

One memory care facility had a sign in the entry inviting male caregivers to a daily 10 a.m. *Men's Coffee* in the room by the coffee shop. I was invited to a weekly evening gathering at

Wealshire called *Wives of the Guys*. It took place after we'd fed our husbands their evening meal. Two women who had lost their husbands at the facility provided a time of informal sharing and encouragement together with light snacks. It was a time to share with those who understood and to be able to laugh together at what our friends and families might not comprehend. The focus was on us as caregivers, not our resident or deceased husbands. Many developed close friendships and continued to attend after the deaths of their loved ones.

Gathering with the *Wives of the Guys* at Wealshire was a time of learning together about dealing with the progression of dementia to death. Those women whose husbands had died shared how the morticians at the facility had a unique tradition of covering the body bag with a 'memory quilt' before leaving the deceased resident's room. It was an alert to the staff that a tribute was about to occur. Allowing the staff and residents to pay tribute was special for them and very meaningful to the family. As snow and the icy winter roads arrived, I reluctantly decided not to drive those twenty miles home late at night.

These types of gatherings are different from having a member of the staff facilitating a group, which becomes more of a sounding board for problems and what the facility can do to improve. At the staff-led groups I attended, staff members would ask about how our loved ones were doing. I sometimes wondered why they had to ask, as though they did not know.

I've learned the importance of seeking support. Support groups, therapy, and connecting with others with similar experiences can be invaluable. Additionally, establishing a network of friends and family who can provide respite and emotional support is essential.

I had continued in the caregiver support group that met virtually during the COVID-19 pandemic, and It was during a regular meeting that another caregiver spoke up, asking if I ever had any plans to harm myself. Though I responded that I didn't, I had given up on finding help after a bad experience with a psychologist who had no idea what dementia was. She blamed me for not communicating with my husband. I was now very resistant to getting any more help or even admitting that I needed help. I was very frustrated and resorted to more late evenings of drinking beer. Loneliness hit hard then, as did guilt and shame. I felt there was no one I could confide in.

As time went by, group members who had recently become widows and widowers would say their goodbyes to our group—yet my husband was still alive. The support group became a misfit for me even though it had been the most significant support in my journey while Louis was at home. There was no other group for this long, unending phase.

However, the acknowledgment of my struggles as our support group met and the inquiries about my well-being were instrumental in helping me confront the challenges I was facing. With the help of the social worker facilitating the group, I managed to enroll for much-needed excellent therapy. Reaching out for help was a challenging step for me, and it was a critical juncture where the involvement of a support group, therapist, and understanding individuals made a profound difference.

I got help from a therapist who was well-experienced in dementia caregiving and assisting caregivers to survive. I knew she had an extraordinary passion for what she did. Her compassionate care has supported me on this journey and reinforced my desire to use what I have learned to help professionals, family, and friends who help caregivers.

During this phase, I realized the importance of having someone nearby willing to listen and provide an outlet for my pent-up emotions. It felt embarrassing, but I had yearned for someone to share my hidden struggles with. I felt they were not something family or friends could comprehend or wanted to hear. I also didn't want to burden them with my struggles, which most of them assumed were over. Those wonderful neighbors of mine were an exception as they invited me over for supper and patiently let me vent my frustrations. They continue to do so, and sometimes, we share meals, often at short notice. I also have the opportunity to drive them to and from the airport when they spend time with their family. To be able to give and receive is a blessing!

Engaging in activities that allowed me to express and process my feelings, such as journaling, meeting with the support group, and with my therapist, were all valuable in navigating the emotional challenges of caregiving. The fear of exploding in public or getting too close to people underscored the importance of seeking professional support and connecting with understanding friends and family members. Human touch and the empathy of those genuinely caring were immensely healing and comforting for me.

Therapy was a lifeline, providing a sense of connection and understanding that was missing elsewhere, ultimately contributing to improved mental and emotional well-being. Having a compassionate, skilled therapist with expertise in dementia caregiving helped me see that reaching out for help wasn't a sign of failure but an act of self-preservation.

Professionals, such as therapists and counselors, can play a pivotal role in supporting caregivers, widows and widowers. Encouraging open communication about struggles and feelings is crucial, even when filled with shame and desperation. Therapy can provide a safe space to address these emotions. I had to recognize that I needed help before it was too late. Having a therapist as the only person to confide in intimately can be especially beneficial when dealing with sensitive or complex issues that may be difficult to discuss with friends or family. Encouraging caregivers to seek help and ensuring that the support systems are in place can make an immeasurable difference in their lives as it has in mine.

I trained and became a facilitator for the Alzheimer's Association. During the pandemic, I had begun facilitating a group of young-onset caregivers and a grief and loss group. I continued with these until I went to graduate school for my Master of Science in Gerontology. I continue to monitor several online groups of widows, widowers, and caregivers of spouses with dementia, and promote groups such as GriefShare to those who have lost a spouse.

Caregivers must be taught self-care techniques and the necessity of seeking early support before they are so overwhelmed that it is challenging to reach them. I had no clue what I needed, which made it hard for anyone to contact me. It turned out that I needed help navigating my collapsing bridge, finding moments of rest and joy, and ensuring the finest care for Louis while protecting his well-being and my own.

Technology

Being a support group attendee using Zoom and facilitating two virtual support groups for the Alzheimer's Association kept me busy during the COVID-19 pandemic. I did not have to carry my distress alone over not seeing Louis during the pandemic, as the support group I was in was not limited only to those caring for a loved one at home. However, having additional informal groups might benefit those with spouses in a memory care facility. Care facilities may appreciate a volunteer to initiate support groups or coffee gathering spots in the facility where family and friends can step away from their loved ones for a break.

COVID-19 provided an incentive for the general public to utilize technology much more than ever before. Telehealth was a unique tool for reaching those who needed care, even without the internet or a computer. If they had cell phone service, a visual telehealth visit with a doctor could now be provided using a GrandPad. These are similar to a cell phone but the size of a tablet and don't need internet access.

Today, the pandemic continues its legacy of virtual technology. There were and still are conferences and seminars I would never have attended in person due to cost, time, and travel, but now I can participate virtually. Webinars and podcasts continue to provide new learning opportunities.

Another aspect I had to consider was that I wished to live independently for many more years. I love my neighborhood and hope to enjoy it for a long time without needing others, including my son, to check on me daily. My search for alternatives started in the times when I felt afraid of Louis while he was still at home, but I was too busy and left the search for later. After hearing about incidents happening to older people in my position, I thought of the stairs in my house.

Like all caregivers, I worried about something happening to me while I was caring for my loved one. What if one day I couldn't get up in the morning? How could our next of kin be told since Louis couldn't use a phone? Now I was worried about how my family and friends would be notified if something happened to me at home. My answer was a free SNUG app at the SnugSafe web site, which I continue to use.

I selected the daily time of 9 a.m., and I get a reminder a few minutes before if I have not checked in by then. Within ten minutes, it alerts two or three people I have named to check on me. It means I don't have to depend on family or neighbors calling me to see if I am okay every day. It is a security blanket both for my family and me.

I wished I had known about GrandPads when Louis was at home struggling to use his phone. Suppose a loved one is placed in a care facility, is alone at home with limited cognitive ability, or is in a rural area without internet access. A GrandPad fills the function of a straightforward cell phone. Family members can set it up to allow calls in and out to family or friends. To make a call, the person using it only has to press a photo or an enlarged name, and the GrandPad also limits who can call the user. Internet browsing can be limited, so if your loved one has Internet access, they cannot place orders or give out credit card or banking information. It eliminates the need to remember names or numbers, and it doesn't require internet or Wi-Fi. The GrandPad also allows you to discontinue a landline to protect the user from strangers, spam, and robocalls. Telemedicine can be used to meet virtually with a doctor or other health professionals.

It looks like a notebook, so even people who have never used a computer or a cell phone can make or receive phone calls or texts. Only those for whom it is set up may call or be contacted, and A GrandPad can also rotate up to two hundred photos so a person in a care facility has a continuous photo show. It gives them a chance to reminisce. For those in the earlier stages of dementia, this resource often provides much pleasure and is something many enjoy sharing with those who visit them. There are other features like games to play. A recent addition similar to Ask Alexa or Hey Google allows the user to ask questions like what day it is or what the weather forecast is. They converse with an owl filled with artificial intelligence!

You can rent a GrandPad on a monthly or yearly basis directly from the company that insures the product, so you do not have to worry if it gets damaged or lost. The monthly or yearly fee comes with excellent customer service if you order it directly from the company. A GrandPad is a beautiful gift for older loved ones with or without disabilities or cognitive difficulties who cannot use a computer or smartphone. It is especially appropriate if you need some control over the phone or internet, such as spending, and want to prevent robo and other calls. There is a product demo you can view at the GrandPad web site. No contract or purchase of the GrandPad is necessary. Advances in technology continue to help with caregiving, and there are a lot of other valuable devices available.

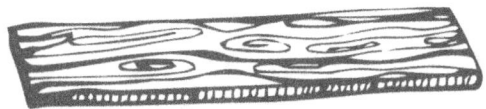

Graduate School

I Am Too Old

It was about four years that Louis had been at the Wealshire of Bloomington, MN, and in and out of qualifying for hospice care at the facility. I was struggling emotionally and physically. My therapist very casually suggested I consider extending my interest in helping caregivers by attending graduate school and obtaining a certificate in gerontology (the study of aging). I felt seventy-two was too old to return to college and was convinced I could never get good grades like the younger students. At first, I thought she was joking! But she wasn't, and I trusted her knowledge–she was also an adjunct professor at a local college. The thought lingered, and I quickly learned that we are never too old to learn. Through that comment, she has helped me use my experiences as a caregiver to find a purpose and fortify my desire to assist others.

Shortly after her suggestion, I did some searching. A call to the University of Minnesota (U of M) about virtual grad school classes in gerontology was a direct line to a gentleman who reinforced that I was not too old to learn. He told me I needed to stay within the state college system for its excellent tuition rates for people my age. The only college with a current virtual gerontology program was St. Cloud. I left a late evening message on the phone at the Gerontology Office at St. Cloud State University (SCSU), giving my age and saying that someone had suggested I apply to study toward a certificate in gerontology. I assumed the response would take several days or that there would be none.

At 8:45 p.m. that same evening, I received a call from Professor Phyllis Greenberg. She asked about my situation and interests. After my response, there was a long pause. I thought I was about to be told I was too old! Then she said, "You're never too old to learn, but I don't think you should go for your certificate; I want you to get your master's with us!"

The campus was closed for the summer, but I did an online summer project with her. Learning the technology was the most challenging part of my first two semesters. The patience of Professor Greenberg and Professor Karasik as I adapted to the technology was fabulous. I managed to start with a 4.0 GPA when I had originally felt I could never compete with younger students.

The college realized the value of virtual technology, which was perfect for me! The best part was that I could attend courses virtually, with the option of driving the sixty-eight miles to campus for one or two in-person classes a month. Evening classes were switched to virtual if the winter roads were questionable.

I went to graduate school while Louis was still in memory care, and eight months after he died, I completed my Master of Science in Gerontology in 2023 at the age of seventy-four. It was an adventure that expanded many of my professional and personal experiences with increased knowledge of aging. Getting my Master's also kept me busy focusing on studying and my determination to succeed.

I have learned more than I ever wanted to know about both dementia and Alzheimer's. I realize that life is too short to dwell on the things that have upset me in the past. I need to go on and figure out ways to love the life God has set before me. It is then that I can share His love with others.

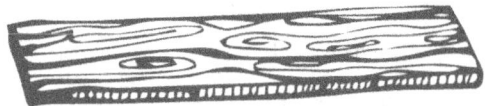

Hospice

Hospice is not something a caregiver can just call in when the caregiving becomes too much to handle at home. It is not twenty-four-hour care and does not include the cost of room and board. I think of approaching hospice as acknowledging the need for comfort of one who is dying and who may be suffering physical and emotional pain rather than the use of possibly painful procedures to extend their life. It is about providing them the most comfort and peace so they are no longer battling pain and can enjoy their final days. It is not a signal to those around you that you have given up.

The first time Louis qualified for hospice care was because of weight loss. A hospice nurse told me to prepare for his life to end in less than four months, though, after two months, he was stable and disqualified from hospice care. Louis lived six more years and qualified for hospice four more times.

Hospice was not ideal, as the first team appeared to lack training with unresponsive residents. For a person with dementia, this was a group of strangers entering his room at Wealshire and trying to handle him with very different care than he was accustomed to. They also did not communicate well with the facility staff.

Louis was still up daily in his wheelchair and fed in the dining area. The hospice team seemed shocked that he was receiving regular meals that were not pureed and that he was not bedridden. Hospice music therapy, which he could not hear, interrupted the everyday routines to which he had become accustomed. One day, a hospice team member came to give him a bath. I intervened, as he had already had his bath two hours earlier. No one from the team had checked his bath schedule.

I was exhausted and desperately needed rest and support from friends at church and my support group, but there was no rest and no time for support. The hospice team expected me to be at Louis' bedside every day, as though he was about to die, and could not understand why I would not be there.

I did not want to face more years of watching Louis deal with his shrinking brain and having no quality of life! He would qualify and start hospice, then be disqualified.

Qualifying was not the hard part; my untold struggle was when he was disqualified, as it meant more unresponsiveness and possible suffering for him. There was simply no way he could tell me of any pain he may have. Each time he no longer qualified, it was as though my bridge had collapsed and the planks ahead were missing. It felt as if I might as well jump into the deep, muddy river below.

Hospice Again and Again

The greatest struggle for me was that Louis qualified for hospice care several times during the six years of memory care, with the first time being after he had been at the facility for less than five months. The third time Louis qualified for hospice, he lasted two weeks before he was considered stable.

I felt anything but stable when, again, his unresponsive state continued. To visit my husband, who had not known me for over three years, had no speech, no hearing, and empty eyes with dilated pupils, was like visiting a post in the center of a parking lot. Louis' life lingered on as I tried to numb my emotions with ineffective coping skills for three more years.

Because his unresponsiveness lasted a total of six years, Louis' case was atypical. It was an agonizing experience of ambiguous loss—that grief without end.

Letting go of a loved one is a complicated and emotional process, as the instinct to provide care and sustenance is fundamental to our human nature. When a patient appears hungry, the natural response is to feed them, regardless of their medical condition. Even when early signs of swallowing difficulties arise, the diet is modified by puréeing food to prevent choking as life is prolonged.

It is essential to have advanced care directives and ensure that medical staff members know the patient's wishes regarding life-sustaining interventions like DNR orders, administering antibiotics, and tube feedings, the latter of which were not allowed at the facility Louis was in. These directives serve as invaluable guidance toward aligning medical care with the patient's values and beliefs.

My husband had not wanted to be kept alive in a vegetative state, but the law states that a person who appears hungry must be fed. Even with POA over his health care, over those slow six years, I couldn't grant his wish not to prolong the vegetative state he was in. Each visit I made became more and more frustrating, though there were no apparent signs of pain until just weeks before his death. A certified nurse's aide (CNA) noticed a grimace while transferring him from his bed to his wheelchair and alerted the nurse. In less than an hour, he was receiving morphine for pain as needed, but since he could not ask, I requested that it be given every three to four hours, which was immediately agreed to.

The decision of whether to prolong life or focus on palliative care is a complex and emotionally charged one. Caregivers, particularly those with POA for health care, often struggle to determine what is truly in the patient's best interest. It's a responsibility that carries a heavy weight, as it involves not just the preservation of life but also the mitigation of suffering and pain. In those last weeks, it was a relief for me to know that Louis would routinely be given pain medication.

It is essential to recognize that the desire to hold on to a loved one is rooted in love and compassion. However, it's equally important to consider whether such efforts prolong undeterminable suffering and pain. The decision to move from aggressive medical interventions to a more comfort-focused approach, such as hospice care, is a profound choice that acknowledges the patient's dignity and seeks to enhance their quality of life during their remaining time.

The decision-making in these situations should be informed, thoughtful, and guided by discussions with healthcare professionals, social workers, family, and, when possible, the patients themselves or the spouse/caregiver. It's an emotional journey marked by difficult conversations and introspection. Ultimately, the goal is to honor patients' wishes and values, providing them with the most compassionate and appropriate care in their unique circumstances.

Caregivers and advocates play a crucial role in facilitating these discussions and decisions, striving to balance preserving life with avoiding unnecessary suffering. It's a profound act of love and responsibility that underscores the complexities of end-of-life care and the importance of respecting individual autonomy and dignity.

Hospice Facts and Who Qualifies

Hospice is a program of care and support for people who are terminally ill. Here are several important facts about it:

- Hospice helps terminally ill people live comfortably.
- Hospice isn't only for people with cancer.
- The focus is on comfort, not on curing an illness.
- A specially trained team of professionals and caregivers care for the 'whole person', including physical, emotional, social, and spiritual needs.
- Services typically include physical care, counseling, equipment and supplies for terminal illness and related conditions, and palliative medication.
- Care is provided in the patient's home or in a care facility and can be two hours a week or more, depending on the condition of the patient.
- Hospice is not simply available full-time to care for a person when a primary caregiver can no longer do so.
- Medicare covers hospice but does not cover room and board for the patient.

See "Hospice Care Coverage" at https://www.medicare.gov/coverage/hospice-care.

People qualify for hospice care if they have Medicare Part A (hospital insurance) and meet all the following conditions.

- The hospice doctor and the regular doctor certify that they're terminally ill with a life expectancy of six months or less.
- Their POA of Healthcare agrees to accept comfort care without any care to cure the illness, like radiation or chemotherapy, that might extend life a little longer, but often with more pain and exhaustion.
- The POA signs a statement choosing hospice care over other Medicare-covered treatments for terminal illness and related conditions.

You can usually get Medicare-certified hospice care in your home or another facility, such as memory care or a nursing home. You may also get hospice care in an inpatient hospice facility. One misconception is that once you cannot care for someone, you should just call hospice. Hospice care is not 24-hour care, and it does not include room and board in a home or a care facility.

See "How Hospice Works" at https://www.medicare.gov/what-medicare-covers/what-part-a-covers/how-hospice-works.

As a primary caregiver, when Louis qualified, I felt I was prepared as I had previously attended some workshops about hospice care. Knowing others who had loved ones in hospice care was helpful, and I always heard the same thing: "Hospice was wonderful."

Only a hospice doctor and the patient's regular doctor or Medicare-qualified doctor can certify that a person is terminally ill and has six months or less to live. As I discovered, the prediction is not always correct, and hospice care can be stopped, extended, or restarted.

The patient pays the deductible and coinsurance amounts for all Medicare-covered services. Health issues that are not part of their terminal illness and related conditions are considered for the comfort of the patient, such as providing oxygen to one struggling with painful breathing. I knew the statement, "Hospice covers everything," was a myth, but not to what extent.

Hospice care was over and above the care at the facility, so the monthly room and board costs did not change. Care varies and can range from just a couple of brief visits each week by a licensed practical nurse (LPN), registered nurse (RN), or certified nursing assistant (CNA) to someone sitting with your loved one in their final hours of life. Hospice care locations differ, ranging from home, assisted living, long-term care facilities, and memory care to special hospice care facilities. Most hospice groups work well with the place they are in and are highly skilled in the terminal condition of the patient. Take into consideration any suggestions made by the facility staff as it is important for them to be able to work well together.

Hospice teams deal primarily with patients in their final days or months of life who have medical issues like terminal cancer. A hospice care team is usually recommended by a care facility, hospital, or medical clinic—whoever deems your loved one qualifies. A significant factor is that caregivers tend to wait too long. Many feel like getting hospice care is admitting that they have given up on extending the life of their loved one. When the moment comes, a caregiver is often so exhausted that they simply go with the recommendation. The facility Louis was in notified me when he qualified. I then filed a request, which was quickly approved, and I notified a hospice team in the area. The first time, I was surprised, as Louis did not seem to be dealing with any physical changes outside of weight loss.

The sudden additional care by a hospice team was a bit massive and overwhelming, given that I did not feel Louis was struggling for life. For people with progressive dementia, strangers coming in and taking them away from regular activities can be very disruptive. Massages might be suitable for those who are dying and alert. However, I question whether they don't just increase anxiety for those in their later stages of progressive dementia. The patient is not familiar with massage and, when in the final stage of dementia, usually cannot tell the therapist what feels good or painful.

Hospice teams are used to dealing with death. As a result, not all hospice teams do well with dementia care because it can be years between the death of the mind and that of the body. To have someone in their care who, after two months, no longer qualifies is not normal for a hospice team.

Louis qualified again for hospice about a year later. We had a different hospice team that I had observed caring for other residents. There was good communication with staff, who helped with his care and did not interrupt the daily routines he was familiar with. This time, it was just a few weeks later that Louis no longer qualified for hospice care.

Having heard how wonderful hospice was for others, I feel it is very appropriate for more sudden losses and those losses from diseases like cancer, where there is often good communication with the patient until the final days before their death. Few hospice groups are trained to handle dementia care involving a patient who has not communicated clearly with anyone for several years.

By the fourth and fifth times my husband qualified, I knew he was getting better care from the current staff in the memory care facility than any hospice group could provide. I did not want that care disrupted by strangers as it could increase his agitation. Our family agreed and decided against more hospice care.

Each time he qualified for hospice, the stress of expecting Louis' death to be imminent was draining emotionally and physically. Friends were unaware of the toll it takes. Preparing for his death and then doing it over and over for six years was emotionally destructive to me. I had made sure I was ready to take care of the remaining payments for our cemetery lots, get notes ready for the mortician, update his obituary, prepare the funeral—Celebration of Life—service as best possible, and arrange for the burial.

Listening carefully to those who had recently lost a spouse was very helpful. Putting messages on my phone when I heard of something else I needed to do when Louis died provided a useful and lengthy list. After three years of disqualifying after qualifying for hospice, I had reached a crisis point with stress, depression, exhaustion, and thoughts of self-harm. I didn't have any strong intent to end my life, but I had no solid motivation to do much else. This was when my binge drinking became a troubling pattern, increasing in both frequency and quantity each time Louis was disqualified from hospice care. Drinking seemed to keep me away from thoughts of harming myself.

Many caregivers find themselves facing a complex web of emotions. Recognizing and addressing these challenges is essential to maintaining well-being and mental health. Feeling hopeless, worthless to society, and untouchable are emotions that can weigh heavily on caregivers.

Final Days of Life

Medical personnel focus on prolonging life for years. Letting go of a loved one is not what family and friends are accustomed to doing. It may be easy to push the person with a terminal condition to try every possible drug or action that causes pain and exhaustion instead of being able to enjoy the little time they have left the best they can. One of the most helpful books I read was *Being Mortal: Medicine and What Matters in the End*. A surgeon, Atul Gawande, shares about caring for his father, who was also a surgeon. He also shares what mattered most to his father at the end of his life. I found the book to be informative on how the dying are treated by those committed to extending life by carrying out painful, devastating procedures that extend suffering. The patient's goals in nearing the end of life are often to be comfortable and be with family and friends where they can still make it a special time without increased pain and suffering.

Deciding not to get a hospice team from outside the facility for the final two times Louis qualified for hospice was a decision I will never regret. The care he received from the dedicated individuals at Wealshire of Bloomington for six years was exceptional. Staff had become a cherished part of our journey and cared for Louis like he was family.

As Louis' final four days came, he could no longer swallow, and he stopped eating. He did not appear in distress because of the morphine he was given. Many of the employees made their heartfelt farewells as our family sat by his bedside. I will forever remember the way they shared many unique and beautiful aspects of my husband's life while they were caring for him, preparing his food, doing his laundry, and so much more, even though he was unresponsive for most of those years. It was an honor to hear from the staff and to realize that the loss to our family was also a profound loss to them. He wasn't just a resident with a dead mind but a unique and cherished human being. This experience reinforced the depth of humanity and compassion that can be found even in the most challenging circumstances.

Early on the morning of August 13, 2022, my journey as a caregiver to my husband came to an end after two decades of caring for Louis since the first signs of cognitive decline appeared. Those initial signs, which I had initially attributed to depression, had been present for several years before a proper diagnosis. It was a journey filled with challenges and sacrifices, but it finally concluded when he passed away at the age of seventy-five. His suffering had ended, and I no longer had to worry that he might be in pain. His death brought me a sense of relief.

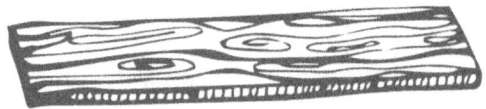

Widowhood

I have crossed my collapsing bridge of caring for my husband with dementia and arrived at a riverbank of widowhood, which has its own challenges. It's a different kind of loss, marked by shifting interests and changes in the dynamics of a marriage of fifty-three years. After making it over a rickety bridge of caregiving, I was in a new chapter of my life. I was alone, as I had been for the past six years, and utterly exhausted.

Even though I had taken the necessary steps to pre-arrange funeral plans—including writing the obituary, planning the funeral service, organizing a lunch, and arranging the burial—these plans were outdated and required additional preparation and meticulous attention to detail. I realize the importance of encouraging family members to pre-plan such events. I also understand the value of flexibility when dealing with the myriad of details that inevitably arise during this emotional and busy time.

In the wake of Louis' passing, there were numerous legal matters to address. I had to sign various documents, notify relevant parties, and change accounts and bills. Removing his name from utility bills, credit cards, and financial accounts proved to be a complex and often daunting task, with most requiring a certified copy of the death certificate, which took about three weeks to receive. It was a process that needed patience and attention to detail while my mind was in a fog.

I discovered the importance of keeping the joint financial account open into which our Social Security benefits were deposited. It was necessary to do so until I received the Social Security death benefit of a surviving spouse and my husband's last month of Social Security benefits had been fully processed. By doing this and waiting three months before I took his name off that account, all was good.

In the United States, you cannot use your spouse's credit cards after they die unless you are a joint account holder. If the account is in your spouse's name alone, using the card is considered fraud—even if you are an authorized user and you have a card with your name on it. I had assumed the card would be frozen immediately and forgot about that. I accidentally used it but was not penalized.

Despite financial details being the last thing you want to deal with at this challenging time, it's also crucial to determine your rights and responsibilities when it comes to your deceased spouse's credit and debit cards. When I finally had Louis' death certificate, I was not prepared for the time each phone call would take. Making those calls and connections took several days. Thankfully, most required only an emailed photocopy of the death certificate, though insurance had stricter criteria. I was able to deal with Medicare online.

I thought the calls regarding Social Security would be the most time-consuming, but there was no wait when I phoned the number the mortuary provided. I only had to verbally verify what the mortuary had already reported. It was terrific to have that call take less than a minute! Their letters of verification and details of the final benefits check were clear, and like Medicare, I could do everything online.

The first year after the death of a spouse is not a time to make big decisions or changes. With the actual passing of my husband came waves of excitement and uncertainty about my future. I found myself in a period of adjustment, learning to navigate a life that was now even more profoundly altered. I finished the two remaining semesters of my Master of Science in Gerontology while building new interests. The caregiving journey has prepared me for many things, but this latest chapter is a path I continue to carve out independently.

Addictions and Suicides Among Older Widows and Widowers

Some distinct challenges and emotions mark the path of widowhood. It's a journey that requires resilience, self-discovery, and a willingness to adapt to new paths in life. However, these can be exceptionally hard to achieve after the failing bridges that caregivers of spouses have had to cross.

Widowed former caregivers struggle with loneliness, isolation, the loss of the job of caregiving, and the loss of social support or meaningful activities. Some are at high risk for suicide (Heuser and Howe 2019), with the highest suicide rate being adults over the age of eighty (Joling et al. 2018). Drug and alcohol addictions are also high among these older people (Han et al. 2019), and rates are highest for those who live alone. Some people die within two years of their spouse's death (Ennis and Majid 2021), and I feared becoming that kind of a statistic.

Older adults may use substances for different reasons than younger adults do, such as to cope with chronic pain, loneliness, depression, anxiety, grief, or stress. They may have various patterns of use, such as binge drinking, prescription drug misuse, or polypharmacy (using multiple medications and supplements).

All of these may result in missed opportunities for screening and the resulting intervention, as few people taking numerous medications and over-the-counter supplements ever request an evaluation from a pharmacist or a primary doctor. Seeing numerous specialists can result in people going to different pharmacies and receiving multiple medicines for one problem. Vitamins, supplements, laxatives, pain meds, fish oil, and other over-the-counter health supplements can be dangerous in combination with prescribed medications. At a recent luncheon with older adults, I recall two people priding themselves on the eight and ten tablets they took with food. They weren't concerned about how the medications interacted because they only cared about what the advertisement said.

Alcohol is the drug most used by older adults, accounting for most admissions to substance use treatment centers in those aged fifty-five and older. The National Institute on Drug Abuse reported in 2020 that about 65% of people aged sixty-five and older report high-risk drinking; that is, exceeding daily guidelines at least weekly in the past year. Furthermore, over 10% of adults in this age group report that they are, in fact, binge drinking, meaning that men consume five or more drinks and women four or more in a few hours (Han 2019). Turning to alcohol to numb emotions can lead to a cycle of dependency, exacerbate feelings of isolation, and deepen the sense of despair.

Potential red flags may include frequent injuries, increased tolerance for other medications, an overabundance of empty beer, wine, or liquor bottles, advanced signs of cognitive impairment (such as forgetfulness, unsteadiness, confusion, memory loss, and slurred speech), symptoms of depression or anxiety, and unpredictable mood swings.

The dark cloud of caregiver depression loomed large on the riverbank of this part of my journey, casting shadows over my resilience and determination. I had left things at home undone. I felt forgotten and unreal. Several times, I felt hopeless, worthless to society, and untouchable, and this was when I attempted to cope with the stress by drinking too much in the evenings. Being retired and alone at home provided the privacy to keep it secret and stay numb with bottled-up emotions. No one seemed to know or care, and it has felt like a brave step to recognize this behavior and consider healthier alternatives. My therapist has challenged me to reach great new heights of living as she has gently guided me over and beyond my darkest moments.

I love dogs and cats and spent lots of time with them on the farm where I grew up. Abby was a great help on my caregiving journey, but she seemed to age much faster once her master was no longer at home. She loved to visit Louis, but sadly, her body finally wore out after Louis no longer knew her and didn't respond to her visits.

Pets are unique, and their presence can help soften the feelings of isolation, contributing to unhealthy coping mechanisms. When older adults need placement in a care facility, finding homes for their pets is tricky. Adopting a senior cat whose owner could no longer keep her has helped me not to feel alone. I now have a cuddly friend named Chatter, who has amazing eye contact and likes to chat with me in kitty language.

I continue to learn from my caregiving journey as my interests and priorities are shifting dramatically. I find plenty to do alone and prefer to avoid crowds. No matter what the season, I enjoy nature and the solitude of the outdoors. I do not miss our retirement plans because we never made any, though we saved for our retirement years. While I was dedicated to Louis' well-being, my passions took a backseat, and as a result, in widowhood, I find I have a renewed sense of self and a desire to explore new interests. This can be both liberating and disorienting as I navigate uncharted territory.

I enjoy writing and finding ways to help current and former caregivers of spouses. My most significant concern is that caregivers get whatever help they need because they may not know how to survive and deal with the emotional, physical, and financial stress of caregiving.

Perhaps, for me, one of the most complex aspects of widowhood following dementia care is the feeling of still, in some sense, being married. The bond forged through our fifty-three years of marriage endures, though the dynamics have shifted. It's a path marked by the profound ache of losing my partner, who was not just a companion but an intrinsic part of my very identity.

As I grapple with the memories and my love for Louis, which remains even in his absence, there's still that feeling of being both connected with and disconnected from the world of couples.

Grief, I've come to realize, is a complex and individual experience that defies neat categorization into stages or any predetermined structure. Just as my husband fought the so-called 'stages of dementia', whether they be three or ten, everyone's grief journey is unique and deeply personal.

The pain of spousal loss is rooted in the loss of intimacy, the absence of the person who knew us like no one else, the ones with whom we shared our hopes, dreams, and the most intimate moments of our lives. While others may empathize and offer their condolences, they can never truly understand the depth of this unique and personal grief.

My grief was so mixed in with trying to accept that I had done my best, but what about that bridge? Could I share how it was collapsing and what I learned so other caregivers could get their own much-needed repairs in the form of help from people who cared? Should I open up about the shame that prevented me from getting help earlier and the unhealthy coping mechanisms I turned to? Would it help anyone? What about the research Dr. Joe Gaugle is doing on the survival of caregivers of spouses? This showed me that as more is understood about how a diagnosis of dementia in their husband or wife affects them, there are people who do care. Research like this begins to help caregivers realize they are not alone. Could we all work together to save the lives of more caregivers?

GriefShare: Grief is Not Something 'To Get Over'

The mission of GriefShare is to equip local churches to mobilize lay ministry teams to help people hurting because of a major life crisis.

I recently completed the excellent thirteen-week GriefShare program for widows and widowers, where attendees were divided into small groups of eight to ten. People stayed in the same group for thirteen weeks, and we had the opportunity to share with those at our table led by a trained facilitator who was also a bereaved spouse. I was reluctant to attend because

I felt I was not dealing with grief anymore, and I did not want to be reminded of the caregiving journey I had been on.

My assumptions were wrong! With a group of three women and seven men, there was laughter as we shared our limited cooking and mechanical skills. As we realized we were not alone, we also shared our feelings of shame for now being able to laugh again, move forward, and enjoy living.

Each week began with a ten-minute review, followed by a fifteen-minute video of how others dealt with various difficulties after a loss. Then, in our groups, for forty-five minutes, we shared our responses. We could also decide not to share and rather listen instead.

GriefShare is a course I highly recommend, and you can repeat it several times if you wish. Not every GriefShare gathering has small table groups, but the small group was the best part for me, so finding out how the course is set up is essential. Knowing I was not alone in some of the shame I was feeling helped me to realize how each person responds differently to a loss. We may feel a sense of relief when a spouse dies, or we may feel intense sadness (Stahl and Schulz 2019). There is also no timeline for grief, and though we will always carry it with us, we will learn how to manage it.

It was at a GriefShare meeting that one person at our table shared how he felt a sense of relief when his wife died, as she was no longer suffering, but that he had felt some shame as others shared their sadness. His words lifted my shame over the relief I felt when Louis died. I had thought I was the only one who felt that way. Sharing feelings can lift us and others as we learn to live alone. In GriefShare, I was challenged to view my journey as a caregiver through a different lens and was given the tools to restore meaning and hope to my life.

To learn I was not alone in the bad coping skills I started when Louis was in memory care and that I continued during his many times of qualifying for hospice was one of the greatest benefits, as I was still struggling with them. Since those thirteen weeks, my moments of guilt and shame have drifted away along with my desire for bingeing.

A Place at the Table (APATT)

I feel blessed to be involved with APATT, which usually meets twice a month on Saturday mornings. All the attendees and leaders have been living in widowhood for a week or two to several years. It is a time of coffee and fellowship, listening to a speaker, and sharing around tables, each one with a group leader.

The total group size varies from sixty to a hundred men and women, hosted by Wooddale Church in Eden Prairie, MN, with attendees from many other churches or without any church connections. The loving care and compassion we all experience there create a special bond of understanding and respect for our uniqueness.

A Place at the Table focuses on the unique needs of widows and widowers in every stage of their journey. Whether you lost your spouse recently, last year or several years ago, APATT has something to offer throughout every phase of your experience:

> **Connection with others:** APATT offers a variety of opportunities for you to connect with others who have experienced a similar loss, from serving together to enjoying coffee and conversation. This can be a powerful source of comfort, understanding, and support.

Spiritual support: APATT offers spiritual support to help you find comfort and strength in your faith.

Education: APATT offers opportunities to learn from speakers and group discussions and find comfort through seminars. This can help you learn how to manage grief and move forward.

Through A Place at the Table, you will make friends with people who understand you in ways others can't. You'll share tears and laughter with people who will make a real and lasting difference in your life and help you keep moving forward in healing and hope.

Praise be to the God and Father of our Lord Jesus Christ, the Father of compassion and the God of all comfort, who comforts us in all our troubles, so that we can comfort those in any trouble with the comfort we ourselves receive from God (II Corinthians 1:3-4).

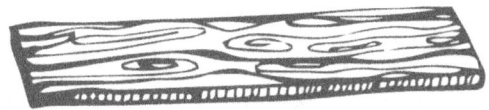

I Have a Purpose

As I stand looking back at the riverbank and the challenging river I've crossed, it's a moment of solitude and reflection. I have traversed my rugged, collapsing bridge and shared my hidden challenges as the supports beneath it began to erode, the gusset plates cracked, and whole planks rotted away.

The solitude here feels different, laden with both loss and the promise of fresh beginnings. The world has shifted significantly during these years. It's a space that feels both isolating and ripe for self-discovery. I have survived an incredible journey.

Since that journey through grief began, I've transformed in countless ways. I'm re-evaluating what holds significance in my life, sifting through the layers of what truly matters. Time has become incredibly precious. My desire to assist other caregivers in navigating similar bridges has intensified. The experience has unveiled capabilities I never knew I possessed. Obtaining my Master of Science in Gerontology has fortified my sense of purpose in assisting those who care for caregivers and helping the caregivers themselves to find mechanisms to survive their journeys in healthier ways than I did.

My social landscape has shifted. After living alone for six years during Louis' time in the memory care facility, the newfound freedom from the immense responsibilities of caregiving is liberating. It allows me to invest time and effort in matters that resonate with me. This freedom propels my desire to support others in similar situations, offering a listening ear and sharing resources that could make a difference. I aim to continue to share what I have learned and to support others as they embark on their challenging journey with a spouse diagnosed with dementia or other lengthy progressive disease.

I enjoy writing, learning new things, and encouraging other caregivers of spouses with dementia by writing responses on blogs and electronic media such as the Alzheimer's Spouse Journal, Dementia Action Alliance, Family Caregiver's Alliance, The Alzheimer's Foundation, Alzheimer's Society of Canada and several other online groups, including support for those of us who are now widows or widowers.

I enjoy working outdoors, listening to the sounds of nature, and feeling the gentle breezes. Experiencing the beauty of a Minnesota winter is as precious as viewing the Northern Lights or sitting on the shore of a lake in the summer, watching the loons raise their loonlets, and hearing their calls at night.

My interests are changing. Volunteer work is a special opportunity to keep my skills from becoming rusty. I am still here for a reason. It is different from the one I envisioned, as I am ready to influence the care of caregivers and those former caregivers who have entered into widowhood.

My greatest wish is that you, who are professionals, friends, or family, will have learned more about what a caregiver may not tell you and more ways to help support them.

If you are a caregiver, always remember you are not alone, even in the toughest aspects of caregiving and during your darkest moments of stress. I hope you have gained helpful knowledge about caring for yourself and being prepared for what lies ahead. I hope, too, that you will feel able to ask for help. We are never too old to learn and we are never too old to help others with what we have learned.

> "God sometimes asks us to abandon the serenity
> of the comfortable and safe
> to walk with Him to one who needs our care."
>
> Jane Grudt

You may contact me at jgrudt@gmail.com I welcome your questions and comments. I'm also available for in-person or virtual speaking engagements.

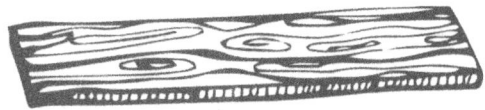

Resources

Differences between Power of Attorney and Guardianship

Power of Attorney (POA)

- **Cost:** The cost of establishing a Power of Attorney can vary but is generally lower than the expenses of obtaining guardianship. You will typically need to pay legal fees to an attorney to draft and execute the POA document.
- **Timeframe:** Setting up a POA is usually quicker than obtaining guardianship. It involves creating a legal document that designates an agent to make decisions on behalf of the principal. This is the person signing the POA, who needs to understand what they are doing by giving another person the power to make decisions on their behalf if they are declared unable to make decisions for themselves.
- **Control:** The principal retains control over their affairs and can choose whom they want to appoint as their agent. This option allows for more autonomy.
- **Flexibility:** POAs can be tailored to specific needs, such as financial or healthcare decisions. If mentally competent, the principal can also revoke or amend them.

Guardianship

A person asking the court for guardianship must first explain what else they tried and why they didn't or won't work.

- **Cost:** Obtaining guardianship can be a more expensive process. It involves court proceedings, legal fees, and ongoing costs associated with the guardian's responsibilities. A guardian can be a relative, another person, or an agency. Anyone can file a petition asking for a guardian to be appointed for an incapacitated adult.
- **Timeframe:** Guardianship proceedings can be lengthy, involving court hearings and evaluations to determine the need for guardianship. The process can take several months or more.
- **Control:** The court appoints a guardian to make decisions for the incapacitated person's personal affairs (medical care, nutrition, clothing, shelter, residence, and safety). A conservator may be appointed to manage their finances, property, and real estate. A person seeking guardianship may be turned down for reasons that may include objections from other family members.
- **Court Oversight:** Guardians are subject to court oversight and may need to provide regular reports to the court, which can add to the ongoing administrative burden and costs. For more information, see https://www.elderlawanswers.com/.

Parts of An Elder Care Legal Plan

- **Durable Power of Attorney of Finances:** A person (the principal) appoints someone to help make financial decisions for them if they should become incapacitated. It allows the appointed person to assist the principal when communicating with banks, insurance companies, and investment firms when they can no longer do so. The power ends at the time of the principal's death.

- **Durable Power of Attorney of Health Care:** The principal appoints someone to help in managing care and treatment decisions when they cannot do so. This appointed person is often a spouse, an adult child, or a trusted close friend. The power ends at the time of the principal's death.
- **Estate Planning:** The process of arranging for the distribution of assets and property *after* death, which may involve wills, trusts, and other legal documents.
- **Guardianship or Conservatorship**: A legal process where a court appoints a guardian or conservator to make decisions on behalf of a person deemed incapable of making their own decisions due to dementia. This process can be far more costly than obtaining a POA while the person can still understand and sign documents. It also requires extensive ongoing financial reports on how all assets, including cash, are used.
- **Living Will:** This is a legal document that outlines an individual's wishes regarding medical treatments and end-of-life care when they can no longer express their preferences. It designates someone to convey their wishes to medical and emergency personnel. Burial preferences can be included.
- **Will:** A legal document that goes into effect *after someone dies*. It does not include any wishes regarding their end of life or immediately after death, such as wishes for burial. It is a tool for when they die that documents to whom they want to direct their money, property, and personal items. *It*

is only effective after death. Any actions listed in it may only be acted on several months after they die.

- **Revocable Living Trust:** A revocable trust allows the owner to alter or cancel provisions while deemed competent. During the life of the trust, income is distributed to the owner. After the owner's death, the property is distributed to the beneficiaries. This document allows flexibility and income; the trust owner can adjust and earn income, knowing the estate will be transferred upon their death.

Comparison of Elder Law Attorneys and Estate Attorneys

Elder Law Attorneys

An Elder Law Attorney addresses the unique legal needs of older adults and their families. They are particularly well-versed in the complex legal issues that often arise as people age. Here are some critical areas of expertise and services provided by Elder Law Attorneys.

- **Power of Attorney:** They can help clients designate someone to make financial and healthcare decisions on their behalf through powers of attorney and advance healthcare directives.
- **Long-Term Care Planning:** Elder Law Attorneys help individuals plan for potential long-term care needs, which may involve strategies to qualify for government benefits, navigate long-term care insurance, or protect some assets from nursing home expenses.
- **Medicaid and Medicare Planning:** They assist clients in understanding and accessing government healthcare

benefits like Medicaid and Medicare, ensuring eligibility and optimizing benefits.
- **Estate Planning:** While similar to Estate Attorneys in this regard, Elder Law Attorneys tailor estate plans to account for the specific needs of elderly clients, such as preserving assets for their care or protecting against financial exploitation.
- **Elder Abuse and Neglect:** These attorneys may handle cases related to elder abuse, financial exploitation, or neglect and advocate for the rights and well-being of elderly individuals.
- **Advance Directives:** They work with clients to create advance directives, living wills, and durable powers of attorney for healthcare that align with their specific healthcare wishes and circumstances.
- **Veterans Benefits:** Elder Law Attorneys assist veterans and their families in understanding and accessing VA benefits that may be available to them.

Estate Attorneys

An Estate Attorney primarily focuses on the legal aspects of an individual's estate planning and the distribution of assets upon death. Here are some critical areas of expertise and services typically provided by Estate Attorneys:

- **Wills and Trusts:** Estate Attorneys help individuals draft wills and establish trusts to dictate how their assets should be distributed among heirs and beneficiaries after their passing.
- **Probate:** They guide families through the probate process, the legal procedure for validating a will, and ensuring the

orderly distribution of assets according to the deceased person's wishes.

- **Estate Tax Planning:** Estate Attorneys assist clients in minimizing estate taxes by employing various strategies, such as setting up tax-efficient trusts and gifting plans.
- **Power of Attorney:** They can help clients designate someone to make financial and healthcare decisions through powers of attorney and advance healthcare directives.
- **Guardianship:** Estate Attorneys may also handle cases related to appointing legal guardians for minors or incapacitated adults.

Medical Terms

- **Advance directive**: A comprehensive document that covers a wide range of healthcare decisions (see Provider Orders for Life-Sustaining Treatment below).
- **Alzheimer's disease:** The most common type of dementia characterized by deteriorating cognitive abilities, behavioral abnormalities, and gradual memory loss. It is one of over 125 diseases that cause dementia.
- **Care advocate:** The primary caregiver of a person who is in a care facility.
- **Care plan**: A personalized document defining the personal, social, and medical needs of a patient or resident, as well as the approaches and interventions that will be taken to meet those needs.
- **Cognitive impairment**: Problems with a person's ability to think, learn, remember, use judgment, and make decisions. Signs of cognitive impairment include memory loss and trouble with concentrating, completing tasks, understanding, remembering, following instructions, and solving problems.

- **Dementia:** A reduction in cognitive function, such as memory loss and other cognitive impairments that affect a person's ability to carry out daily tasks.
- **Geriatrician**: A doctor with advanced training in the identification, management, and care of elderly persons, including those with dementia.
- **Gerontology:** The study of aging.
- **Home health care:** Nursing care, therapy, and personal help. It may include non-medical services offered to people in their homes.
- **Hospice:** Comfort care without curative intent; the patient has chosen not to pursue treatment because the side effects outweigh the benefits. Hospice care requires two physicians to certify that the patient has less than six months to live if the disease follows its usual course. Hospice does not cover room and board in a care facility or a patient's home, nor is it 24-hour care unless or until deemed necessary. The care can take place wherever a patient calls home. Minnesota law does not allow or authorize euthanasia, suicide, or assisted suicide. State law requires that oral food and water be given to a patient who accepts them. Relief of pain and control of suffering must be offered.
- **Life-sustaining treatment (life support):** Any treatment intended to prolong life without curing or reversing the underlying medical condition. This can include mechanical ventilation, artificial nutrition, and hydration.
- **Long-term care (LTC):** When someone with a chronic illness, such as dementia, cannot carry out everyday tasks independently, they need LTC, which includes services and assistance in a nursing home or memory care facility.

- **Neuropsychological assessment**: A thorough assessment of cognitive and psychological functioning frequently used to determine the diagnosis and course of dementia.
- **Palliative care:** A holistic approach to medical care that focuses on improving the quality of life for people suffering from life-threatening conditions such as dementia. Palliative care is comfort care with or without curative intent.
- **Provider Orders for Life-Sustaining Treatment** (POLST): While an Advance Directive is a comprehensive document that covers a wide range of healthcare decisions, a POLST form is focused on end-of-life decisions that require immediate medical attention and is portable so it can be with the patient. For instance, it may specify whether you want to receive cardiopulmonary resuscitation (CPR), antibiotics, or be put on a ventilator. Different states may refer to it by a variation of the term:

    POLST or POST (physician/provider orders for life-sustaining treatment).

    MOLST (medical orders for life-sustaining treatment).

    COLST (clinician orders for life-sustaining treatment).

    MOST (medical order for scope of treatment).
    - https://polst.org/state-polst-programs/
    - www.mnpolst.org (State of Minnesota)

A Successful Support Group

- is a group of people supporting and encouraging each other as they face common issues
- is well-facilitated by a knowledgeable, compassionate professional

- ensures that what is shared stays in the group, is confidential, and is not shared with others
- has time for sharing divided as equally as possible
- allows everyone an opportunity to share every time
- has excellent attendance by all caregivers
- provides information about resources and coping mechanisms
- offers advice on what lies ahead
- provides help for dealing with family members
- is limited to caregivers of people with a common issue
- is a haven for sharing true feelings
- meets weekly or twice a month, usually with three to twelve caregivers
- has a facilitator who listens and takes up very little of the group time
- has a facilitator who understands that caregivers need the opportunity to support other caregivers, as it gives them a sense of purpose
- doesn't include speakers because they take time away from caregivers with topics that are not of interest to all
- welcomes laughter with other caregivers as a stress release
- does not tell caregivers what they already know or repeatedly shame them with, "You need to take care of yourself."
- affirms for each caregiver that they are doing their best and attending the group to make their best efforts better

Steps for Caregiver Support

- **Seek professional help.** Consult with mental health professionals specializing in caregiving-related issues. They can provide guidance, coping strategies, and emotional support tailored to your needs.

- **Join support groups.** Consider joining support groups for caregivers during and after your caregiving journey. When appropriate, join a group of widows and widowers. These groups offer a sense of community and a safe space to share experiences and emotions.
- **Build a social network.** Cultivate relationships with friends and family who understand your challenges and are willing to provide emotional support. Don't hesitate to reach out and express your needs. Respect that not everyone will comprehend your needs or be comfortable knowing how to help.
- **Have a list of ways people can help you.** Email it to those who offer to help and give a date and time, such as, "Jack has a dental appointment on (day) and (time) for about one hour at (place)," or, "Jack needs a haircut this week. If you could take him, it would give me time to get groceries."
- **Meals**. "Having lunch together on any Tuesday at (place) and splitting the bill would be great." Be prepared with a list of favorite foods or carry-out meals like burritos.
- **Prioritize self-care.** Make self-care a priority in your life. Engage in activities that bring you joy and relaxation, and be mindful of your physical and mental well-being.
- **Educate others.** Share your experiences and insights with others to raise awareness about caregivers' challenges, help reduce stigma, and encourage support.
- **Advocate for resources.** Become an advocate for more resources, services, and policies that support caregivers and address their unique needs.

- **Encourage early intervention.** Encourage caregivers to seek help and support early in their caregiving journey rather than waiting until they are in crisis.
- **Remember, seeking help is a sign of strength, not weakness.** By addressing your emotional well-being and supporting others on their caregiving journeys, you can contribute to a more compassionate and supportive caregiving community.
- **Find a grief group without a time limit for grieving.** We learn that grief is not something we ever get over. Our grief often begins once it appears our spouse no longer recognizes us, and during the in-between time until the death of the body, it can be very difficult to find support or feel a part of any group. It is often the most stressful period of grief for the caregiver.

Memory Care Planning Assistance

- medicaidplanningassistance.org is a free service provided by the American Council on Aging.
- The American Council on Aging offers current information on Medicaid eligibility in each state and also helps with qualifying. They provide a free, fast, non-binding Medicaid long-term care eligibility test at https://www.medicaidplanningassistance.org/medicaid-eligibility-test/.
- For "Answers to All of Your Questions About Medicaid Long Term Care," see their FAQs at https://www.medicaidplanningassistance.org/medicaid-long-term-care-faq/. There are also pages of information about eligibility for each state, which changes yearly. This website has excellent information for those with minimal assets and income.

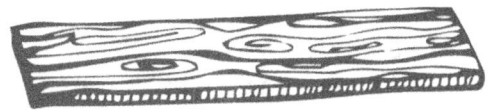

References

Boss, P. (2011). Loving someone who has dementia: How to find hope while coping with stress and grief. John Wiley & Sons. https://doi.org/10.1002/9781119438519.ch88

Ennis, J., & Majid, U. (2021). "Death from a broken heart": A systematic review of the relationship between spousal bereavement and physical and physiological health outcomes. *Death Studies*, *45*(7), 538–551. https://doi.org/10.1080/07481187.2019.1661884

Gaugler, J. (Director). (2023, November 6). *A New Era: Understanding Lecanemab, Donanemab, and Emerging Therapies for Alzheimer's Disease* [Webinar]. https://www.youtube.com/watch?v=DUtQq9Aa3WU

Gaugler, J. E., Jutkowitz, E., Peterson, C. M., & Zmora, R. (2018). Caregivers dying before care recipients with dementia. *Alzheimer's & Dementia: Translational Research & Clinical Interventions*, *4*(1), 688–693. https://doi.org/10.1016/j.trci.2018.08.010

Gawande, A. (2014). Being mortal: Medicine and what matters in the end. Metropolitan Books.

Han, B. H., Moore, A. A., Ferris, R., & Palamar, J. J. (2019). Binge Drinking Among Older Adults in the United States, 2015 to 2017. *Journal of the American Geriatrics Society*, *67*(10), 2139–2144. https://doi.org/10.1111/jgs.16071

Harel, D., Band-Winterstein, T., & Goldblatt, H. (2022). Between sexual assault and compassion: The experience of living with a spouse's dementia-related hypersexuality—A narrative case-study. *Dementia, 21*(1), 181–195. https://doi.org/10.1177/14713012211032068

Heuser, C., & Howe, J. (2019). The relation between social isolation and increasing suicide rates in the elderly. *Quality in Ageing and Older Adults, 20*(1), 2–9. https://doi.org/10.1108/QAOA-06-2018-0026

Joling, K. J., O'Dwyer, S. T., Hertogh, C. M. P. M., & van Hout, H. P. J. (2018). The occurrence and persistence of thoughts of suicide, self-harm, and death in family caregivers of people with dementia: A longitudinal data analysis over 2 years: Suicidal thoughts in family caregivers of persons with dementia. *International Journal of Geriatric Psychiatry, 33*(2), 263–270. https://doi.org/10.1002/gps.4708

Leggett, A. N., Sonnega, A. J., & Lohman, M. C. (2020). Till death do us part: Intersecting health and spousal dementia caregiving on caregiver mortality. *Journal of Aging and Health, 32*(7–8), 871–879. https://doi.org/10.1016/jagp.2018.01.097

Minnesota Dept of Public Health. (2017). *Minnesota Provider Orders for Life-Sustaining Treatment (POLST)*. www.mnpolst.org (State of Minnesota). https://mn.gov/emsrb/assets/POLST%20Form_MN_FINAL%202017-03.13_tcm21-283534_tcm1116-368779.pdf

Stahl, S. T., & Schulz, R. (2019). Feeling relieved after the death of a family member with dementia: Associations with post bereavement adjustment. *The American Journal of Geriatric Psychiatry, 27*(4), 408–416. https://doi.org/10.1016/j.jagp.2018.10.018

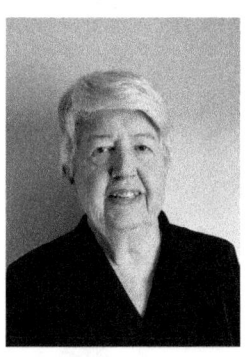

About the Author

JANE enjoys writing and helping those who care for caregivers. She is a registered nurse with a master of science in gerontology and worked nights in a nursing home, followed by many years as an office manager.

Caring for her husband with Alzheimer's disease was a role that threatened to overwhelm her with untold struggles of shame and embarrassment. When no longer a caregiver at home, she facilitated two Alzheimer's Association support groups prior to obtaining her Master's. She loves the outdoors and prefers snow blowing and tree trimming to cooking and housework. She lives in Minneapolis, MN. Contact: Jane Grudt at jgrudt@gmail.com

> "God sometimes asks us to abandon the serenity
> of the comfortable and safe
> to walk with Him to one who needs our care."
>
> Jane Grudt

www.ingramcontent.com/pod-product-compliance
Lightning Source LLC
LaVergne TN
LVHW021343080426
835508LV00020B/2093